Comments on *Kidney Failure Explained* from readers

'I was so impressed by the wonderful way the book is presented, in terms which everyone can understand. Our committee has recommended the book to our members.'
Roy Bradbury, Chairman, Sheffield Area Kidney Association

'This is a very well written book and it should be of great value to renal patients.'
Professor R Wilkinson, Consultant Nephrologist, Freeman Group of Hospitals, Newcastle-upon-Tyne

The book is excellent and will prove very valuable to a variety of different groups. I shall certainly be recommending it to patients and to general practitioners in particular.'
Dr Robin Winney, Consultant Renal Physician, Department of Renal Medicine, The Royal Infirmary of Edinburgh

'The content of the book was realistic but positive and covered all aspects of kidney failure. I have already started recommending it to some of my patients.'
Ros Tibbles, Pre-dialysis Sister, Department of Renal Medicine and Transplantation, the Royal Hospitals NHS Trust

'*Kidney Failure Explained* not only answered all the questions I wanted to ask, it also answered a lot of questions I hadn't even thought of. Books of this kind are badly needed. Thank you for a clear and precise text, in language I can understand.'
Dennis Jackson, CAPD patient

Printing history
First published 1999
Printed with revisions 2000

The authors and publishers welcome feedback from the users of this book.
Please contact the publishers.

Class Publishing, Barb House, Barb Mews, London W6 7PA, UK
Telephone: (020) 7371 2119
Fax: (020) 7371 2878
email: post@class.co.uk
http: www.class.co.uk

A CIP catalogue record for this book is available from the British Library

ISBN 1 872362 90 7

Designed and illustrated by Darren Bennett

Edited and typeset by Ruth Midgley

Indexed by Jill Somerscales

Production by Landmark Production Consultants Ltd, Princes Risborough

Printed and bound in Slovenia by printing house Delo Tiskarna by arrangement with Korotan Ljubljana

KIDNEY FAILURE EXPLAINED

Everything you always wanted to know about
dialysis and kidney transplants
but were afraid to ask

Dr Andy Stein, MRCP
Consultant Nephrologist, Walsgrave Hospital, Coventry

Janet Wild, RGN
former Educational Services Manager, Baxter Healthcare Renal Division

CLASS PUBLISHING • LONDON

FOREWORD 1

As someone with End Stage Renal Failure, I have tried to find out as much as I can about my disease. Many of the books I tried were either out of date, too technical or just plain dull.

This book is different. It deals with the issues patients want to know about and does so in a way that is clear and understandable but not superficial.

Each chapter is clearly identified and contains all the information anyone could want – 'Kidney Failure Explained' answers everything you always wanted to know about dialysis and transplantation but were too afraid to ask.

And why shouldn't you be? Learning for the first time that you have kidney failure can be a traumatic experience not only for the patient but also for family and friends. The treatment is lifelong and complex, often including a bewildering array of drugs, diets and other strict regimes.

I've found that having the right information at the right time is vital – it has given me some sense of control and helped me to cope.

I believe Dr Andy Stein and Janet Wild's excellent book should be read by every kidney patient and their family. I can recommend it without hesitation.

Austin Donohoe
Chairman, National Kidney Federation

FOREWORD 2

For most patients medicine is a very confusing subject, with a totally different and at times apparently alien vocabulary. To complicate matters further, within medicine there are numerous specialities, each dealing with a separate organ or system within the body, and with a different group of individuals caring for that speciality. Renal medicine, or nephrology as it is often called, has more than its share of confusion. Add to that the words 'kidney failure' and it is not surprising the alarm that this creates for our patients. The complexities regarding the causes of kidney disease, its complications, and the different methods of treatment, all potentially lead to further confusion and concern.

It is appropriate and timely that a book should have been written to clarify this situation. Dr Andy Stein and Janet Wild are to be complimented on their achievement. This book is written with the patient's welfare as its first priority and succeeds in this regard. The various chapters clearly explain the subject matter and should help patients with kidney disease to understand their problem – or at least to ask the appropriate question to the appropriate person. Especially useful is the glossary of terms used in nephrology, to be found at the end of the text.

It is a pleasure to be asked to write this foreword and I would recommend this book to all kidney patients, new or old, as standard reading.

John Walls, Professor of Nephrology,
Leicester General Hospital.

INTRODUCTION

This is a book about kidney failure. It has been written primarily for people with kidney failure. But, as any partner, friend or family member of a kidney patient knows, kidney failure is a family business. 'They' also usually want to know as much as possible (sometimes even more than the patient) about the disease. So, this book is also for 'them', the silent support that keeps a kidney patient alive.

The idea for this book came at the end of a dinner I had with a group of twenty or so peritoneal dialysis patients in 1995. I had gone away with them on an 'adventure weekend' to North Wales. It was a dark and blustery winter's night. At the end of the meal, I asked them what they hated most about kidney failure. I expected answers like: 'the arrogance of the doctors', 'having to take Calcichew tablets', 'the never ending drudgery of doing four peritoneal dialysis exchanges every day'.

I was wrong. The patients all said that the worst thing was the 'lack of information on kidney failure'. I knew I could give them what they wanted. So, that night, I promised them that I would write them a book describing all aspects of kidney failure. They said they wanted a book that was understandable, hard-hitting and truthful. They didn't want to be patronised. They didn't want wool pulling over their eyes. If kidney failure was to kill them, they wanted to know, and when, and why.

So, I make no apologies to those kidney patients who 'don't want' to know. I believe that they are only a small proportion of the total, and that they probably will not buy this book anyway.

The book would never have come to fruition without my co-author, Janet Wild, who has many years' experience as a senior kidney nurse. Janet and I have written 11 out of the 15 chapters, the other four being written by friends of ours, all of whom currently work in kidney medicine: Gemma Bircher, Peter Ellis, Jean Hooper and Ian Lawrence.

As in all aspects of medicine, different doctors favour different ways of treating patients. I have tried to present the views of the majority in this book. I have also tried to point out controversial areas – either where we don't really understand things (for example, why kidneys fail in the first place) or where there are real differences of opinion (such as which treatment is 'the best', or when a treatment is available in one kidney unit but not in another). The limitations of the treatments currently available is one of the themes of the book.

Over the last two years, whenever I was meant to be writing my thesis or a scientific paper to further my own career, my mind turned back to that dark night in Wales. And my computer somehow drew me to fulfil my promise. Here it is.

Andy Stein

ACKNOWLEDGEMENTS

Kidney disease is about teamwork. This book could not have been written without the combined efforts of the following people. Professor Gerry Coles (Cardiff), inspired Andy Stein to be a kidney doctor, for which he is thanked. Professor John Walls (Leicester) and Professor Terry Feest (Bristol) were the first doctors to review the book and both devoted much time to improving it. Subsequently the book was also reviewed by Dr Gillian Matthews (Andy Stein's mother), Dr Steve Nelson (St George's, London) and Dr Phin Kon (King's, London). The guest writers, Gemma Bircher (Leicester), Peter Ellis (King's, London), Jean Hooper (Gloucester) and Dr Ian Lawrence (Leicester), all took to their task keenly and with speed. Individual chapters were reviewed by Mr Paul Gibbs (King's, London), Dr John Cunningham (The London), Professor Mike Nicholson (Leicester), Dr Ian Abbs (Guy's, London), Mr Geoff Koffman (Guy's, London) and Dr Roger Greenwood (Stevenage).

The early force behind the book was Val Said, a kidney patient, who works tirelessly as a volunteer advocate for patients with kidney failure in the UK. Her efforts have been subsequently supported by Austin Donohoe, the Chairman of the National Kidney Federation.

We are grateful to Saheed Rashid (Baxter Healthcare), Saima Butt (Roche Pharmaceuticals), Sally Taylor and Mike Stark (Janssen-Cilag) and Tim Proger (Kimal) for raising funds for the book.

The publisher, Richard Warner, insisted on literary excellence but never 'pushed' us faster than we could cope with. Darren Bennett is thanked for his clear diagrams and design. Lastly, and most importantly, we thank Ruth Midgley, the editor, for insisting on factual accuracy and clear writing for our readers. She converted this book from something that was 'alright' to something about which we are proud.

DEDICATION

This book is dedicated to the tens of thousands of patients with kidney failure in the UK. Their will to live has inspired us all.

CONTENTS

1 WHAT IS KIDNEY FAILURE?

2 TOXIN 'CLEARANCE'

3 FLUID BALANCE

4 Blood pressure

5 Anaemia and erythropoietin

6 Renal bone disease

7 Dialysis – the basics

8 Peritoneal dialysis

9 HAEMODIALYSIS

Chapter contributed by Peter Ellis, Research Nurse, King's College Hospital, London

10 TRANSPLANTATION

11 BLOOD TESTS

12 DIET

Chapter contributed by Gemma Bircher, Chief Renal Dietitian, Leicester General Hospital

13 PSYCHOLOGICAL ASPECTS

Chapter contributed by Jean Hooper, Clinical Psychologist, Gloucester Royal Hospital

14 SEXUAL PROBLEMS

Chapter contributed by Dr. Ian Lawrence, Consultant in Diabetes and Endocrinology, Leicester Royal Infirmary

15 THE TREATMENT SHORT-FALL

1 What is kidney failure?

This first chapter begins by describing the kidneys and how they work. Then it explores what goes wrong when someone has chronic kidney failure, what causes this problem and why it should be treated.

Introduction

Chronic kidney failure is a serious, long-term medical condition. At the present time, there are approximately 30,000 people in the UK who are either on dialysis or who have received a kidney transplant to treat chronic kidney failure. This is approximately one person in 2,000, making it a very rare condition. This means that a typical family doctor will have only one kidney patient 'on their books'.Chronic kidney failure has many possible causes, but the effects are usually the same. The kidneys become less and less able to do their normal work. After a time, the kidneys stop working almost completely – a condition called end-stage renal failure (ESRF), end-stage renal disease (ESRD) or end-stage kidney failure. Treatment that takes over the work of the patient's kidneys is then essential. The main treatments are dialysis – either peritoneal dialysis (PD) or haemodialysis – and transplantation. These treatments cannot 'cure' kidney failure but they can improve health and prolong life.

Kidneys – what and where are they?

Most people have two kidneys. These important body organs are shaped like beans and are 12 centimetres (about 5 inches) long, which is about the length of your palm. They are 6cm wide and 3cm thick. Each kidney weighs about 150 grams (about 6 ounces). The kidneys lie under the ribs at the back, just above the waist, one on either side of the body (see *diagram* on next page).

The kidneys' main job: making urine

The main job of the kidneys is to make urine. Blood is pumped by the heart to each kidney. The kidneys 'sieve' this blood and make urine from it. Each kidney has a drainage system that takes urine from that kidney to the bladder. This drainage system is like a funnel with a tube (the ureter) that connects the funnel to the bladder (see *diagram* on next page). Urine passes down the ureters (one for each kidney) into the bladder. Urine is stored in the bladder before being passed from the body via another tube, called the urethra. The bladder holds about 400 ml (about 3/4 pint) of urine when 'full'. People normally pass about 2 litres of urine per day.

Location of kidneys and urinary system

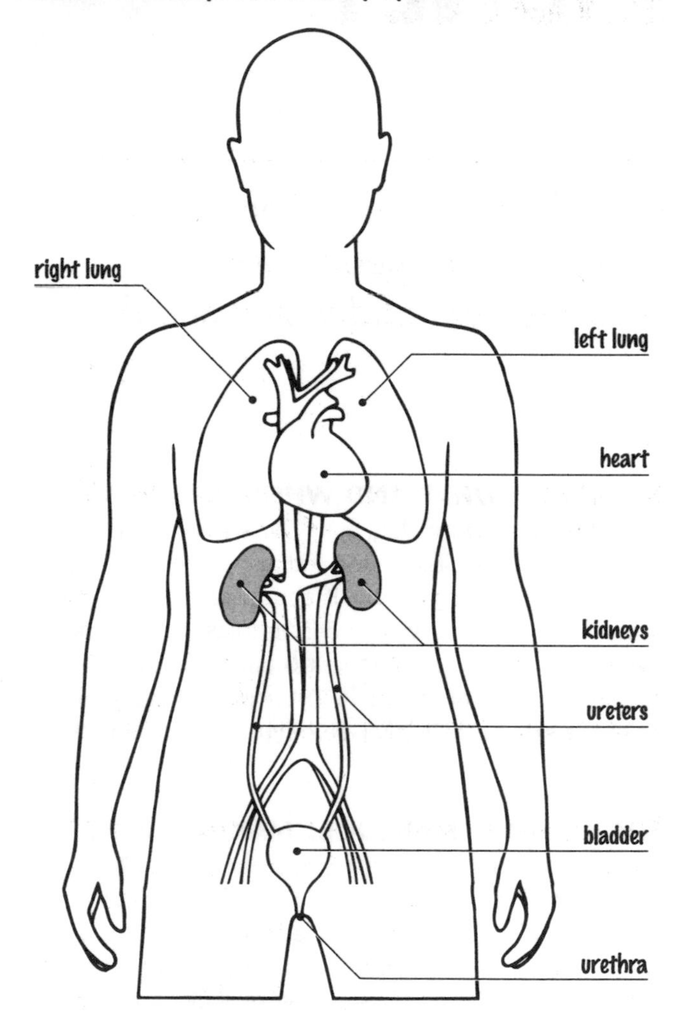

WHY MAKE URINE?

The kidneys make urine in order to perform their two most important functions. These are:

1. Removing toxic wastes from the blood – a process called 'clearance'. (See *below* for a brief description, and *Chapter 2* for more details.)

2. Removing excess water from the body – a process called 'ultrafiltration'. (See *page 3* for a brief description, and *Chapter 3* for more details.)

REMOVING TOXIC WASTES

The kidneys play a very important role in getting rid of the waste products of food. The food that we eat is normally digested in the stomach and the bowels. During digestion, the food is broken down into simple substances that can be carried around the body in the blood. These 'good things' in the bloodstream provide every part of the body with the energy it needs for work, and with the substances it needs for growth and repair.

When the different parts of the body make use of the various 'good things' in the blood, they also produce waste products. These wastes are toxic (poisonous) to the body and make people unwell unless they are removed. Like the 'good things', these 'bad things' also travel around the body in the bloodstream.

When the waste products of food reach the kidneys, it is the job of the kidneys to get rid of them in the urine. What the kidneys do is to sieve and filter the blood, removing the wastes and putting them in the urine, but leaving the 'good things' in the blood. Healthy kidneys generally have no problems getting rid of all the many toxins normally produced by the body.

In people with kidney failure, however, the levels of toxins build up in the blood. It is this build-up of toxins that makes people with kidney failure feel unwell. When someone is in the early stages of kidney failure, there are usually no symptoms, because the toxin levels are not high enough to cause them. (This can be true even when the kidneys are working at less than 25% of their normal capacity).

A kidney

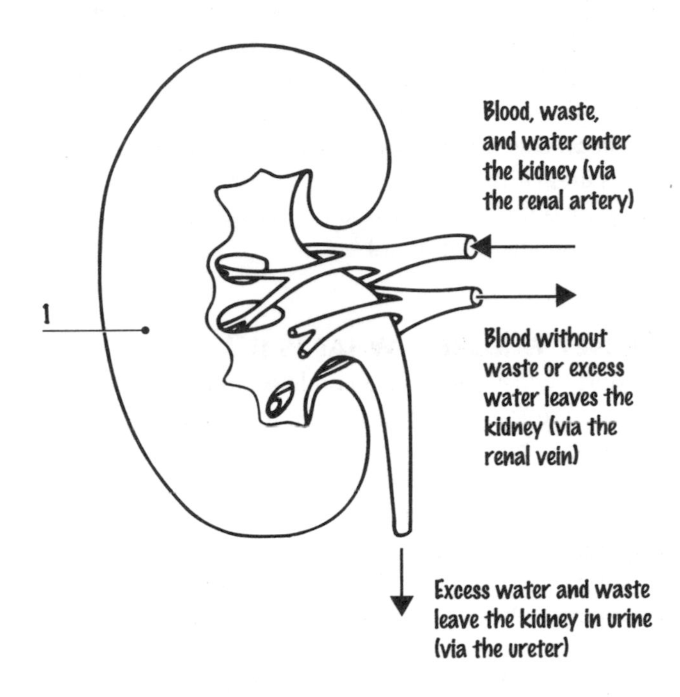

1 In this part of the kidney there are 1,000,000 filtering units (nephrons)

REMOVING EXCESS WATER

The second most important function of the kidneys is to remove excess water from the body. As well as getting rid of the waste products of food, healthy kidneys also remove excess fluids from the body. Like the food that we eat, the water (and tea, coffee, beer and all other liquids) that we drink is digested in the stomach and bowels and absorbed into the blood. When the blood reaches the kidneys, the normal sieving and filtering process removes any excess water and puts it in the urine. So, normal urine contains not only the waste products of food, but also any excess water that has been drunk.

In people with kidney failure, water cannot so easily be put into the urine. Excess fluid can therefore build up in the body, causing it to become 'waterlogged' – a condition called fluid overload (see *Chapter 3*). This may lead to swelling of the ankles, and shortness of breath due to excess fluid in the lungs.

A kidney filtering unit (nephron)

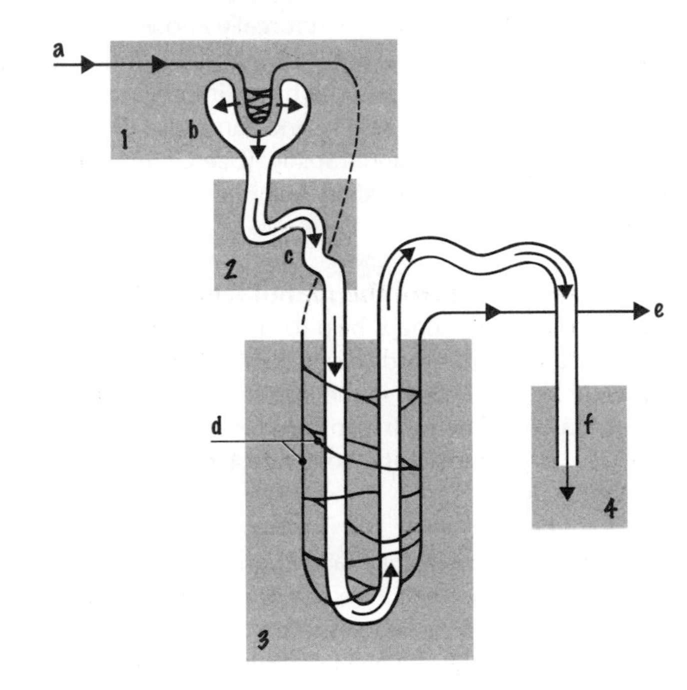

1 Blood from the renal artery (a) is filtered inside a glomerulus (b)

2 Water and waste products filtered from the blood enter a tube system (c)

3 Blood vessels (d) take most of the water back around the body via the renal vein (e)

4 Waste products and excess water (the urine) are removed via a drainage duct (f) that eventually drains into the bladder

OTHER FUNCTIONS OF THE KIDNEYS

As well as making urine to perform their two main functions (removing toxic wastes and removing excess water), the kidneys have three important 'extra' functions. These are:

1. Helping to control blood pressure. The blood pressure is usually finely controlled by the kidneys. When someone's kidneys fail, their blood pressure usually goes up, although it is not really known why. High blood pressure does not usually cause symptoms unless the pressure gets very high, but it increases the risk of a stroke or heart attack, and can cause the kidneys to deteriorate more rapidly. (See *Chapter 4* for more information about kidney failure and raised blood pressure.)

2. Helping to control the manufacture of red blood cells. The kidneys help to control the manufacture of red blood cells in the bone marrow. The red blood cells float in the liquid part of the blood (called plasma). Their job is to carry oxygen around the body. Every part of the body needs oxygen to function properly.

When someone has kidney failure, they make fewer red blood cells than normal. As a result, most people with kidney failure become anaemic (i.e., they are short of red blood cells). This anaemia contributes to the tiredness suffered by most people with kidney failure – it is not only high toxin levels that cause tiredness. (See *Chapter 5* for more about anaemia and how it can be treated.)

3. Helping to keep the bones strong and healthy. Calcium and phosphate are two minerals found in the blood and in the bones. If the bones are to stay strong and healthy, there must be a correct balance of these minerals in the body. The kidneys help to maintain this balance. When someone develops kidney failure, the normal balance between calcium and phosphate in the body is lost. The level of calcium in the blood goes down, while the level of phosphate in the blood goes up. Unless this imbalance is treated, it will result in a condition called renal bone disease. This may cause aches and pains in the bones, and even fractures. (See *Chapter 6* for more information about renal bone disease and its treatment.)

KIDNEY FAILURE – WHAT IS IT?

In short, kidney failure is a condition in which the kidneys are less able than normal to perform their usual functions. These functions are:

- removing toxic wastes;
- removing excess water;
- helping to control blood pressure;
- helping to control red blood cell manufacture;
- helping to keep the bones strong and healthy.

This book is about the long-term condition known as chronic kidney failure or chronic renal failure. (There is also another condition, known as acute kidney failure, in which the kidneys suddenly stop working. Short-term treatment may be needed for acute kidney failure, but the kidneys usually get better on their own. This book does not tell you about acute kidney failure.)

When someone has chronic kidney failure, the kidneys become less and less able to do their work. This happens gradually, usually over a period of many years. Eventually, the kidneys stop working almost completely – a condition called end-stage renal failure or ESRF. Treatment is then essential to take over the work of the kidneys and so keep the patient alive. The treatments for ESRF are dialysis – either peritoneal dialysis (PD) or haemodialysis – or a kidney transplant.

WHAT ARE THE SYMPTOMS?

In the early stages of chronic kidney failure, there are often no symptoms. Later, the condition may cause any of the following:

- itching;
- weakness or tiredness;
- loss of appetite;
- poor concentration;
- restless legs;
- leg cramps;
- swollen ankles;
- shortness of breath;
- poor sleeping;
- poor sex drive;
- feeling cold.

HOW IS KIDNEY FAILURE DIAGNOSED?

The only reliable way to diagnose kidney failure in the early stages is by measuring the levels of a substance called creatinine in a patient's blood. Creatinine is one of the many waste products that build up in the blood when someone has kidney failure.

Creatinine levels are measured by a simple blood test. The higher the creatinine level, the worse is the kidney function. The normal level of creatinine is between 45 and 120 μmol/l (micromoles per litre of blood). If a patient's creatinine is over 120 μmol/l, then they have kidney failure (see *Chapter 2* for more details). As soon as the creatinine level starts to rise, the kidney problem is already serious. Creatinine levels slightly above normal (say, 150 μmol/l) may mean that the kidneys are already down to about 75% of normal function.

Creatinine testing is used not only to detect kidney failure, it is also used at all stages of kidney disease – before dialysis, during dialysis, and after a transplant. The amount of creatinine in the blood is the single most important piece of information that doctors and nurses require when looking after people with kidney failure. (See *Chapter 2* for more information.)

WHAT CAUSES KIDNEY FAILURE?

There are hundreds of different diseases that can cause chronic kidney failure. Usually, however, the condition is due to one of the following:

1. Nephritis. The term nephritis covers a group of conditions in which there is long-term inflammation of the kidneys ('neph-' means 'kidney', and '-itis' means 'inflammation'). Sometimes the condition is described, more specifically, as glomerulonephritis or GN ('glomerulo-' refers to the glomeruli, which are part of the kidneys' filtration unit).

The causes of most types of nephritis are unknown. Nephritis can only be diagnosed for certain by a kidney biopsy. This involves removing a small piece of kidney with a hollow needle so that it can be examined under a microscope.

2. Polycystic kidney disease (PCKD). This is an inherited disease (a disease that runs in families) in which both kidneys become filled ('poly-' means 'many') with cysts (abnormal lumps). If someone has PCKD, they will have a 50% chance of passing the problem on to each of their children.

PCKD is diagnosed by ultrasound (an investigation that uses sound waves to produce a picture of the kidneys). Polycystic kidneys, though abnormally large because of the cysts, do not work well. Most people with PCKD eventually develop ESRF.

The cysts in PCKD can remain a problem after treatment for kidney failure has started. A cyst can burst, bleed or get infected – any of which may cause pain. Occasionally, a large cyst that is particularly troublesome will have to be drained through a long, hollow needle, or removed by an operation. Sometimes, people with polycystic kidneys have to have one of them removed to make room for a transplanted kidney.

3. Pyelonephritis. 'Pyelo-' refers to the drainage system of the kidney (it looks like a funnel) and '-nephritis' means 'kidney inflammation'. So, pyelonephritis means 'inflammation of the kidney drainage system'. Pyelonephritis is diagnosed by ultrasound, or by a special X-ray of the kidneys called an intravenous pyelogram or IVP, for which an opaque dye is first injected into the bloodstream.

Pyelonephritis can sometimes be linked to repeated kidney infections. These may have gone undetected for many years, perhaps having occurred in childhood.

Pyelonephritis is sometimes caused by a condition called reflux nephropathy (or 'reflux'). In this condition, a valve where the ureter enters the bladder (*see diagram, page 2*) is faulty. This faulty valve allows urine from the bladder to flow back up the ureter to cause problems in the kidney.

4. Renovascular disease. As people get older, their arteries tend to become 'furred' up with cholesterol and other fats. Smoking makes this process occur at a younger age. This 'furring up' (which is called atheroma or atherosclerosis) gradually narrows the arteries (the blood vessels that take blood from the heart to every part of the body).

Atheroma in the arteries that supply the heart's own muscle leads to angina and heart attacks. If the atheroma affects the arteries that supply blood to the brain, it may cause a stroke. Atheroma can also affect the arteries that supply blood to the kidneys, the renal arteries. This is called renovascular disease ('reno-' means kidney, and '-vascular' means blood vessel). Renovascular disease is a particularly common cause of kidney failure in older patients.

5. Diabetes mellitus. Whether diabetes is controlled by insulin, tablets or diet, it can cause kidney failure. This happens most often when people have had diabetes for longer than ten years. By this stage, they are also likely to have other long-term complications of diabetes, such as heart disease or eye problems. Diabetes is the commonest cause of kidney failure in many parts of the UK, accounting for 40% of dialysis patients.

6. Unknown. In about 30% of patients with ESRF, the cause of the kidney failure is never discovered. This is because the kidneys often appear small and shrunken when shown by ultrasound. For this reason, a diagnosis of 'two small kidneys' is often made. 'Two small kidneys' really means that the kidneys are small, but doctors don't know why. It is presumed that 'something' happened to the kidneys years ago, and they have slowly shrivelled up since.

THE 'PROGRESSION' OF KIDNEY FAILURE

When chronic kidney failure is still at an early stage, most patients feel quite well. This is because their failing kidneys 'overwork' to keep the levels of body wastes normal. This hides the fact that the kidneys are failing. In other words, the kidneys have a lot 'in reserve'. The body manages for quite some time to adapt to high levels of toxins and water in the blood. It does this by making the kidneys work harder.

The rate at which kidney failure gets worse varies from patient to patient. Also, the symptoms that patients get when they have similar levels of kidney function can vary considerably. Some patients get symptoms when their kidney function is 90% of normal, whereas others do not get symptoms until their kidney function is down to 1% of normal!

However, for most people with kidney failure, the following description will apply:

- When kidney function is 75% of normal, the blood creatinine (see *Chapter 2*) may be 150 µmol/l, and the patient feels fine.
- Most patients only start to feel unwell when their kidney function is down to about 10% of normal, and their blood creatinine is about 500 µmol/l.
- When kidney function is down to about 5% of normal, the blood creatinine may be over 800 µmol/l, and most patients feel very unwell. Dialysis or a transplant is then needed.

If someone has chronic kidney failure – whatever its cause – their kidneys will eventually very probably stop working completely. Doctors do not know why failing kidneys almost always get worse, or why people with chronic kidney failure almost always progress to ESRF.

WHAT IS ESRF?

End-stage renal failure or ESRF is considered to begin when treatment by dialysis or a transplant becomes essential to keep the patient alive. When kidneys reach 'end-stage', they very rarely get better. Once someone develops ESRF, they will always have it, even after they have had a transplant.

If the kidneys start to fail in an older person (say, in someone over 70 years old), that person may live out their natural lifespan without experiencing any problems from their kidneys. This is because the kidneys can take up to 10 years to progress to ESRF. So, sometimes, older people never need treatment for their kidney failure. However, when someone over 70 does need treatment for kidney failure, they will be given it.

HOW IS ESRF TREATED?

ESRF can be treated by dialysis or by a kidney transplant. It is usual for a patient to undergo a period of dialysis before transplantation is considered. Dialysis and transplantation provide alternative ways of taking over the work of the patient's failed kidneys.

1. Dialysis. In this treatment, some of the work of the kidneys is performed by artificial means. (See *Chapter 7* for a description of what dialysis is and how it works.) There are two main types of dialysis: peritoneal dialysis (PD) and haemodialysis. (PD is described in detail in *Chapter 8,* and haemodialysis in *Chapter 9.*) Either PD or haemodialysis usually provides about 5% of the function of two normal kidneys.

2. Transplantation. This treatment involves the removal of a normal kidney from one person (the donor), and its insertion into a patient with kidney failure (the recipient). Transplantation is done by a surgeon during a transplant operation. A 'good' transplant provides about 50% of the function of two normal kidneys. (Transplantation is described in *Chapter 10.*)

WHEN SHOULD DIALYSIS BE STARTED?

Dialysis is usually started either when:

- a patient has severe symptoms of kidney failure which affect normal daily life; or
- the levels of toxins and/or water in the body are so high that they become life-threatening.

A blood creatinine level of 800 µmol/l is generally taken to indicate the onset of ESRF. However, the actual level varies from patient to patient (see *Chapter 2*). Most doctors now usually try to start patients on dialysis when their blood creatinine level is about 600 µmol/l (i.e., just before the onset of ESRF). However, individual decisions always take into account more than just creatinine levels.

CAN THE NEED FOR DIALYSIS BE DELAYED?

Once a patient has developed ESRF, dialysis should be started at once. However, if someone with chronic kidney failure has not yet developed ESRF, it may sometimes be possible to delay the need for dialysis.

The following treatments may delay the need for dialysis in some patients:

1. Treatments to control blood pressure. High blood pressure is known to speed up kidney failure. Doctors therefore make great efforts to keep the blood pressure of their kidney patients normal. Keeping the blood pressure really low (consistently 130/80 or less) can delay the need for dialysis by years. This is true for all patients with kidney failure – the cause of the kidney failure makes no difference. (See *Chapter 4* for more about blood pressure and kidney failure.)

2. Treatments to suppress the immune system. When kidney failure is due to nephritis (see *page 5*), the need for dialysis can sometimes be delayed by tablets called immuno-suppressants. In some types of nephritis, the body's immune system (the system that normally fights infection or foreign objects in the body) starts to attack the patient's kidneys and stops them working properly. So, tablets that dampen down the immune system – such as the steroid tablet called *prednisolone* – can be used to treat the kidney problem. In some patients, such treatments are very successful, and return the kidney function to normal or near normal. In other patients, these tablets are less successful. Even so, they may delay the need for dialysis by many years. (There is more information on the immune system in *Chapter 10,* the chapter about Transplantation.)

3. Use of ACE inhibitors. This is a more controversial treatment that may delay the need for dialysis in some patients. Some people with kidney failure (especially kidney failure caused by nephritis) have a large amount of protein in the urine. Normally there is next-to-no protein in the urine. If a kidney patient has a raised level of protein in the urine, doctors often attempt to reduce it with a type of blood pressure tablet called an ACE inhibitor. Whether this treatment in fact delays the need to start dialysis is unproven.

WILL DIALYSIS OR A TRANSPLANT SOLVE THE PROBLEM?

Neither dialysis nor a kidney transplant can 'cure' a patient with chronic kidney failure. These treatments can control the symptoms of kidney failure, but they cannot get rid of the symptoms completely nor restore the kidneys to health.

1. Dialysis. When someone is treated by dialysis, the symptoms of kidney failure never really go away completely. This is because either type of dialysis – PD (see *Chapter 8*) or haemodialysis (see *Chapter 9*) can provide only about 5% of the function of two normal kidneys. So, when a patient starts dialysis, they will usually have only about 10% of the function of two normal kidneys (5% from dialysis, and 5% from their own kidneys). This is simply not enough.

The symptoms of kidney failure will also tend to worsen if there is under-dialysis – i.e., if insufficient dialysis is given to bring the amount of creatinine in a patient's blood down to target levels (see *Chapter 2* for more information).

Even though dialysis technology has its limitations, it does exist and it does work. So it is sensible to start treatment as early as possible – before a patient becomes very unwell. This means that some patients may feel relatively well when they start dialysis. The doctor will be able to tell from a patient's blood creatinine and symptoms when is the best time to start dialysis.

2. Transplantation. A kidney transplant is more effective than dialysis at removing the symptoms of kidney failure. This is because a transplanted kidney can provide up to 50% of the function of two normal kidneys. However, transplants have their own problems. They do not last for ever and it may be necessary for a patient to have a second transplant or to resume dialysis. (See *Chapter 10* for more information about transplantation.)

WHY TREAT KIDNEY FAILURE?

If someone with ESRF is not treated by dialysis or a transplant, they will develop severe kidney failure symptoms (see *page 5*), and then, after a few weeks, they will die.

Given the terrible result if no treatment is given, it may seem stupid to ask: 'Why treat kidney failure?' The answer seems obvious – 'to keep patients alive'. To a certain extent this is true. When people have ESRF they will die without treatment.

So, yes, the main purpose of the treatment of ESRF is to keep patients alive. However, there is little point in keeping patients alive if their quality of life is so poor that they don't want to be alive.

There are, in fact, several reasons why treatment is given to patients with kidney failure. Firstly treatment prolongs life, but it also aims to make patients feel better, and to return them to a good quality of life. To achieve this, the two main functions of the kidneys – removing toxins (see *Chapter 2*) and maintaining the body's fluid balance (see *Chapter 3*) – have to be performed for the patient. Dialysis and transplantation can perform both these vital functions.

KEY FACTS

1. The two main functions of the kidneys are:
   - removing toxic wastes;
   - removing excess water.
2. Kidney failure is a condition in which the kidneys are less able to carry out these two functions.
3. Whatever the original cause of kidney failure, it tends to get worse over a period of years.
4. A blood test (the creatinine level) is used to measure the amount of work that the kidneys can still do.
5. Most people with chronic kidney failure develop a condition called end-stage renal failure (ESRF).
6. ESRF can be treated by dialysis or (usually better) by a kidney transplant.
7. For most kidney patients, good control of blood pressure is the only way to delay the onset of ESRF and the need for dialysis.
8. The treatment of kidney failure (by dialysis or transplantation) is effective, but it is not a 'cure' and may not get rid of all the symptoms.

2 TOXIN 'CLEARANCE'

This chapter looks at ways of measuring the ability of the kidneys (or dialysis) to remove ('clear') toxins from the blood.

Introduction

One of the main functions of the kidneys is to remove the toxic waste products of food from the blood. This function is sometimes called 'clearance', because toxins are 'cleared' away. When someone has kidney failure, their kidneys become less efficient at clearing waste products from the blood. This leads to a build-up of toxins in the blood. It is this build-up that makes people with kidney failure feel unwell. Doctors do not know which particular toxin or toxins make people ill.

Why is clearance measured?

Tests that indicate the clearance of toxins from the blood are extremely important when someone has kidney failure.

Clearance measurements are used:

- in the diagnosis of kidney failure;
- to assess the severity of kidney failure;
- to decide whether it is time for a patient to start treatment by dialysis;
- to monitor treatment by dialysis;
- to assess how well a transplant is working.

Clearance provides a more reliable guide to a kidney patient's condition than is possible from either a physical examination or from an account of the patient's symptoms. Some patients get a lot of symptoms when their kidney function is not too bad. Others get few or no symptoms even when doctors and nurses think that they need dialysis.

How is clearance measured?

There are tens of thousands of different substances in the blood. Fortunately, there is no need to measure most of them. The overall ability of the kidneys to clear wastes from the blood is assessed by measuring the blood levels of two particular substances. These are called urea and creatinine.

Urea is a waste product produced by the liver. When we eat protein (such as in meat and eggs), the body uses this protein to repair itself and to build muscles. The 'used' proteins (now in the form of substances called amino acids) are taken in the blood to the liver, where they are changed into urea. The urea then travels in the blood to the kidneys, where it enters the urine.

Creatinine is a substance created by the muscles whenever they are used. The harder our muscles work, the more creatinine they produce. This is a little bit like a car engine producing exhaust fumes. So, our muscles are like the engine which drives the car, and creatinine is like the exhaust from the engine. Like urea, creatinine is carried in the blood to the kidneys, where it enters the urine.

Creatinine production

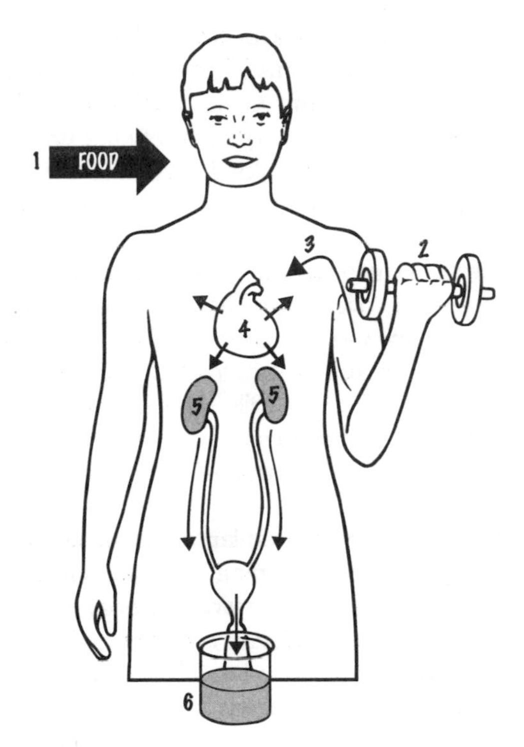

1 Protein is eaten in food
2 Protein is used to make strong muscles
3 Creatinine is produced in the muscles when they are used
4 Creatinine is pumped around the body in the bloodstream by the heart
5 Blood is filtered in the kidneys
6 Creatinine is passed in urine along with other waste products

Why measure urea or creatinine?

Normal healthy kidneys can remove both urea and creatinine from the body quite well. However, when someone has kidney failure, the blood levels of both these substances rise above normal.

- **The normal blood level of urea** is between 3.3 and 6.7 mmol/l (millimoles per litre of blood).
- **The normal blood level of creatinine** is between 45 and 120 µmol/l (micromoles per litre of blood).

Urea and creatinine are not themselves particularly harmful to the body. Creatinine is not even a toxin. However, tests that indicate the clearance of urea and creatinine from the body, provide an indication of the clearance of all the thousands of harmful toxins that are produced by the body. In kidney failure, there is a build-up of urea, creatinine and all these toxins.

A substance which is known to indicate the presence of another substance is called a 'marker'. Urea and creatinine do not themselves make people with kidney failure feel ill. However, both urea and creatinine are markers for the many more harmful toxins that do make kidney patients feel unwell.

Types of tests

Different tests show how well or badly the kidneys (or dialysis or a transplanted kidney) are managing to clear the blood of urea or creatinine.

There are basically two types of tests:

- **blood tests,** which measure the levels of urea or creatinine in the blood (see *page 12*); and
- **clearance tests**, which measure the amount of urea or creatinine removed from the blood (see *page 14*).

BLOOD TESTS FOR UREA OR CREATININE

Blood tests provide a direct measurement of the levels of urea or creatinine present in a patient's blood. These levels can then be compared to normal levels (see *page 11*), or to a range of expected or target levels at different stages of a patient's illness or treatment (see *page 13*).

In simple terms, the higher the levels of urea or creatinine in a patient's blood, the worse the kidney (dialysis or transplant) function. The lower the levels, the better.

In fact, the picture is not quite so simple. Blood urea tests are not always a reliable guide to a patient's kidney function. This is because blood urea levels are affected by things other than the kidneys, such as the amount of protein in the diet. Blood creatinine tests are a generally more reliable guide to kidney function, and have now largely replaced blood urea tests.

It is also the case that blood levels of both urea and creatinine are affected by an individual's overall size and muscle bulk. Larger and more muscular people have higher blood levels of creatinine and urea than smaller and less muscular people. This is true both when someone is healthy and at all stages of kidney failure. Overall size and muscle bulk must therefore be taken into account when looking at an individual's blood urea and blood creatinine test results.

BLOOD CREATININE BEFORE DIALYSIS

Blood tests that measure the level of creatinine in a patient's blood provide doctors with the information they need to decide:

- whether a patient has kidney failure; and
- how bad it is.

The normal level of creatinine in the blood is known to be between 45 and 120 μmol/l. So, if anyone has a creatinine level of over 120 μmol/l, it means that they have kidney failure.

The normal level for any particular individual depends on their overall size and muscle bulk. For example, a healthy large man can be expected to have a normal blood creatinine of 120 μmol/l (at the top of the normal range). However, the same blood creatinine of 120 μmol/l in a small woman might indicate the start of kidney failure. Her normal blood creatinine might be as low as 45 μmol/l (at the bottom of the normal range).

At the start of kidney failure, blood creatinine levels tend to increase slowly over time. This can take months, or, more often, many years. However, when the kidneys have almost completely failed, the blood creatinine level rises more rapidly. Patients will probably feel unwell when their creatinine level gets to more than about 500 μmol/l, equivalent to about 10% of normal kidney function.

At all stages of kidney failure, large patients will have a relatively higher blood creatinine level than small patients. So, for example, a large man whose kidney function is only 25% of normal could have a creatinine level of 400 μmol/l. A small woman who has 25% of normal kidney function could have a creatinine level of 250 μmol/l.

STARTING DIALYSIS

Dialysis is usually started when a patient's blood creatinine is between 600 and 800 μmol/l. A level of 800 μmol/l is equivalent to about 5% of the function of two normal kidneys. Unless someone with kidney failure starts dialysis at this point, they will become very unwell.

The actual creatinine level at which any patient starts dialysis will take into account their size and muscle bulk.

General guidelines are based on the needs of an 'average' person. However, most people are not average. So, the precise creatinine level for starting dialysis is different for different patients.

BLOOD CREATININE DURING DIALYSIS

Measurement of blood creatinine continues to be important after a patient has started dialysis. This applies to patients on either type of dialysis – peritoneal dialysis (see *Chapter 8*) or haemodialysis (see *Chapter 9*).

Blood creatinine levels provide vital information about how well dialysis is working. A 'high' level of creatinine could mean that a patient is not getting enough dialysis – i.e., dialysis is not removing enough toxins.

When planning an individual patient's treatment, doctors and nurses aim to keep the patient's blood creatinine at or below recognised 'target' levels. These targets take into account both the size of the patient and the type of dialysis.

The following table summarises the target creatinine levels for different sizes of patient:

Weight	Target creatinine
Less than 60 kg	Less than 600 µmol/l
60 to 90 kg	Less than 800 µmol/l
More than 90 kg	Less than 1000 µmol/l

A blood creatinine of 800 µmol/l is the accepted target level for a person of average size and muscle bulk. This target applies all the time for average-sized peritoneal dialysis (PD) patients, and before dialysis for average-sized haemodialysis patients:

PD patients. The blood creatinine of a PD patient remains almost constant. This is because PD patients have dialysis treatment every day. Their treatment therefore aims to keep the creatinine permanently below 800 µmol/l.

Haemodialysis patients. The blood creatinine of a haemodialysis patient does not stay at a constant level. Patients on haemodialysis usually have treatments three times each week. This means that their blood creatinine rises in the days between dialysis sessions, and falls during dialysis. The goal is to keep the creatinine below 800 µmol/l before dialysis, and below 300 µmol/l after dialysis. In other words, a haemodialysis session should cut the creatinine level by two thirds, at least.

The fact that the creatinine target levels are the same for PD and haemodialysis (before dialysis) indicates that the two techniques provide roughly the same amount of dialysis. One is not 'better' than the other.

If dialysis does not achieve creatinine target levels over a period of time, the patient will be in danger of redeveloping the symptoms of kidney failure. This problem is called under-dialysis.

Under-dialysis is corrected by increasing the amount of dialysis. Ways of doing this are described in later chapters (see *Chapter 8* for PD, and *Chapter 9* for haemodialysis).

BLOOD CREATININE WITH A TRANSPLANT

Ideally, the blood creatinine of an average-sized person with a transplanted kidney should be less than 120 µmol/l (i.e., the upper limit of normal). However, even if a transplant is working well, the blood creatinine may not return to normal levels. A creatinine level of below 200 µmol/l is generally considered satisfactory for a patient in this situation.

If a transplanted kidney starts to fail, the patient's blood creatinine level will rise again. When it exceeds 600 µmol/l, it is probably time to start dialysis again. The creatinine level for restarting dialysis is therefore the same as the level at which a patient who is new to kidney failure would start on dialysis. This is because the period in which a transplant fails is very similar to the period before dialysis is first started.

UREA OR CREATININE CLEARANCE TESTS

Many renal units now use tests called urea or creatinine clearance tests in addition to blood tests for measuring their patients' kidney (dialysis or transplant) function.

Urea or creatinine clearance tests are sometimes preferred to simple blood tests because they link the amount of urea or creatinine in a patient's blood to the size of the patient's muscles. In some situations, this may make these tests a more reliable measure of the severity of a patient's kidney failure.

The test used to measure the clearance of urea is called urea kinetic modelling (or UKM). The amount of urea clearance is expressed in terms of Kt/V (pronounced 'K...t...over V'). (See *Chapter 9* for more details.)

The clearance of creatinine is measured in millilitres per minute (ml/min) or litres per week (l/wk).

- **The normal creatinine clearance level** is about 120 ml/min or 1200 l/wk.

This means that you 'clean' all the blood in the body about 35 times a day. The fact that 120 is the normal level of urea and creatinine clearance and also the upper limit of normal for blood creatinine is a coincidence.

Blood tests measure the levels of toxins remaining in the blood. So, when blood urea or blood creatinine are measured, the lower the number the better. High numbers reflect poor kidney (dialysis or transplant) function.

The opposite is true for urea and creatinine clearance measurements. This is because clearance tests measure the amount of toxins removed from the blood. So, for clearance test results, the higher the number, the better. A low number indicates poor functioning of the kidneys (dialysis or a transplant).

When the blood creatinine is down to 800 µmol/L (at the onset of ESRF), the creatinine clearance is usually down to about 5 ml/min (i.e., about 5% of normal).

Dialysis provides about 5 ml/min of creatinine clearance (i.e., about 5% of normal). So, when a patient starts dialysis, the combined efforts of the kidneys and dialysis is only about 10% of what two normal kidneys can do. This is why patients with kidney failure rarely feel perfectly well on dialysis. Neither PD nor haemodialysis is good enough at clearing toxins.

HOW IS CLEARANCE MEASURED?

Different methods for measuring the clearance of urea or creatinine are used for different patients, depending on their type of treatment.

Patients not on dialysis. Clearance of urea or creatinine in these patients (either pre-dialysis or with a transplant) is measured by comparing:

- the amount of urea or creatinine passed in the patient's urine over a period of 24 hours; with
- the amount of urea or creatinine in the patient's blood.

To provide accurate results, it is essential that the collection of urine is done very carefully. Otherwise, the information will be less reliable than that obtainable from simple blood urea or blood creatinine tests.

PD patients. The method used for measuring clearance in PD patients is much more accurate than that for non-dialysis patients. In PD patients, clearance is measured by comparing:

- the amount of urea or creatinine in 24 hours' worth of the patient's used dialysis fluid (and also in the urine that they might pass); with
- the patient's blood urea or creatinine level (taking into account the patient's size).

Haemodialysis patients. Clearance can also be accurately measured in haemodialysis patients. For haemodialysis patients, the method is to compare:

- the patient's blood urea or blood creatinine level before dialysis; with
- the patient's blood urea or blood creatinine level after dialysis.

When measuring clearance in dialysis patients it is also necessary to take into account the urea or creatinine passed in any urine, as well as patient size. Urine production dwindles, making it necessary to increase the amount of dialysis about one year after starting dialysis.

Urea or creatinine clearance during dialysis

When monitoring urea or creatinine clearance in a dialysis patient, doctors and nurses will compare that patient's levels with generally accepted levels for patients on dialysis. The current guidelines state that:

PD patients should have:

- a creatinine clearance of 70 l/wk; and
- a urea clearance (Kt/V) of 2.0/wk.

Haemodialysis patients should have:

- a creatinine clearance of 100 l/wk; and
- a urea clearance (Kt/V) of 1.2 for each dialysis session.

These goals are the same for all patients – as they take into account size and build, as well as the amount of waste that patients can get rid of through their own kidneys.

Key facts

1. Creatinine and urea are two waste products that are normally passed in the urine.
2. The levels of urea and creatinine in the blood are an indication of how well the kidneys (or dialysis or a transplant) are working. Blood creatinine levels are a more reliable guide than blood urea levels.
3. The higher the level of urea or creatinine in the blood, the worse the kidney (dialysis or transplant) function. Generally speaking, the lower the numbers, the better.
4. Larger people may have higher blood creatinine levels than smaller people because they have bigger muscles.
5. Urea and creatinine clearance may be more accurate ways of measuring the efficiency of dialysis. This is because these tests take each patient's body size into account.
6. The higher the urea or creatinine clearance, the better the kidney function. So, the higher the clearance numbers, the better.
7. Kidney function usually deteriorates with time, making it necessary to increase the dialysis dose.

3 Fluid Balance

This chapter describes how the amount of water in the body is controlled by the kidneys. It looks at the problems of too much or too little water in the body and gives information on how to deal with them.

Introduction

One of the two main functions of the kidneys is to remove excess water from the body. Water comes into the body from drinks, and also from food, especially high-liquid food such as soup, jelly and ice-cream. By removing excess water from the body, the kidneys are able to control the body's water content. This is called fluid balance. To understand fluid balance, it helps to know a bit about what the body is made up of.

Flesh and fluid

The body is made up of two main parts: flesh and fluid. The flesh is all the solid parts of the body, such as bone, muscle and fat. Most of the fluid part is simply water, such as the water in blood, urine and saliva. Men have approximately 60% of fluid to 40% of flesh in their bodies, whereas women, whose bodies contain a higher proportion of fat, have approximately 55% of fluid to 45% of flesh (see *diagram*).

The easiest way to see a change in the amount of fluid in the body is to measure body weight. The known weight of 1 litre of water is 1 kilogram. So, if a person weighs themself, then drinks 1 litre of water and then re-weighs themself, their weight will show an increase of 1 kilogram.

Fluid and flesh proportions in the human body

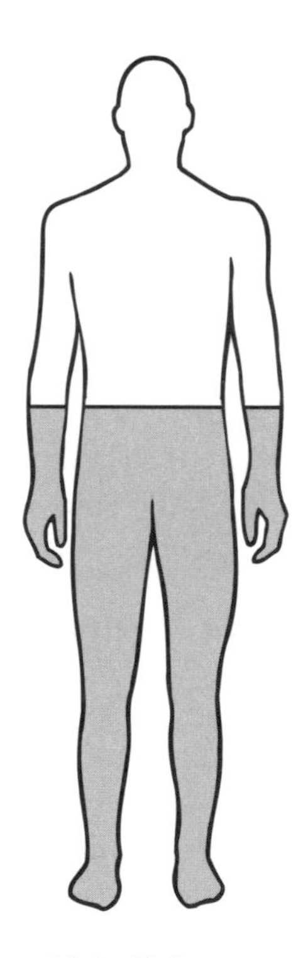

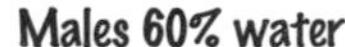

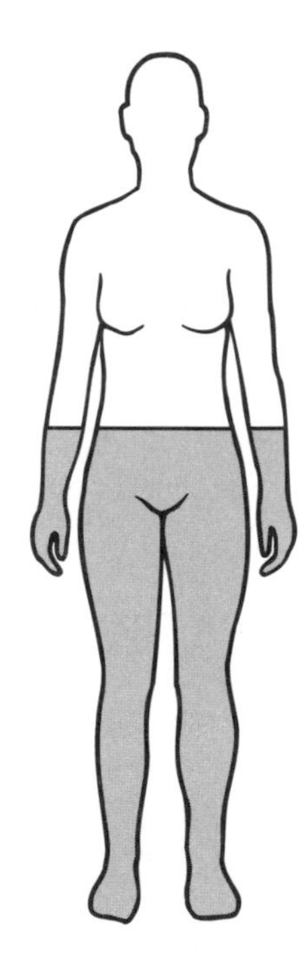

What is the 'target weight'

The term 'target weight' means the weight that the doctor considers to be the 'best' weight for an individual patient. At this weight, there will be neither too much nor too little water in the body. Men will have about 60% fluid to 40% flesh, and women about 55% fluid to 45% flesh. A kidney patient's target weight may go up or down as flesh weight may be gained or lost. Flesh weight increases if someone eats too much, or may decrease due to dieting or illness.

Control of fluid balance

Normal healthy kidneys can control the amount of water in the body with ease. If you do not have kidney failure, you do not have to think about your fluid balance. This is because your kidneys control the amount of urine you pass.

Water loss from the human body

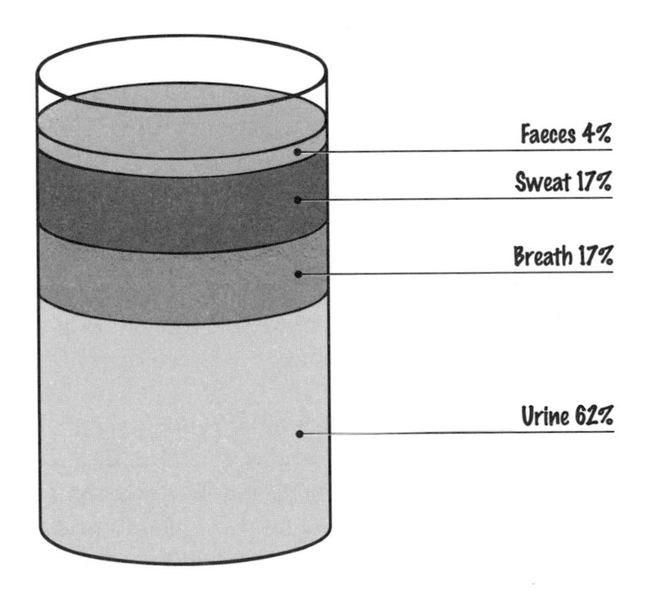

If someone drinks ten pints of water (or beer), they will usually pass about ten pints of urine. Similarly, if they drink three cups of tea per day, they can expect to pass the equivalent of about three tea cups of urine.

Fluid is also lost from the body in other ways – as you breathe, when you sweat and in your faeces (see *diagram*). If someone becomes very hot, they will sweat more. To control fluid balance, they will then need to compensate for the sweat losses by passing less urine.

In kidney failure, it is different. Many kidney patients do not pass any urine at all. Others pass exactly the same amount of urine every day, no matter how much they drink. This means that these patients are unable to control how much water is in the body. If someone with kidney failure drinks too much, they may keep that fluid in their body. This is called fluid overload (see *below* for more details). Conversely, if someone with kidney failure drinks too little, or loses too much water from the body (say through sweating), they will become dehydrated (see *page 18*). Finding the balance is not easy.

Sodium and fluid balance

Sodium is a mineral that plays a part in helping control the body's fluid balance. Table salt contains sodium, and dialysis patients are sometimes asked to reduce the amount of salt in their diet. This is because salty foods, such as crisps and many processed and tinned foods, make people thirsty. If people with kidney failure drink too much, they may develop fluid overload.

What is fluid overload?

This is a condition in which there is too much water in the body. It is caused by drinking too much fluid, or not losing enough. Fluid overload often occurs with high blood pressure (see *Chapter 4*). By and large, high blood pressure does not cause any symptoms.

When the water content of the body reaches a very high level, excess water collects under the skin. The problem usually first shows as swelling around the ankles. This is called ankle oedema. The reason the ankles are affected first is simple – gravity tends to make fluid fall to the bottom of the body.

If fluid overload is not treated, the swelling due to excess fluid slowly creeps up the body into the thighs, and then into the lower abdomen and lower back. Hopefully, by this stage, the patient will have asked for medical help. If not, fluid will continue to spread up the body, and eventually settle in the lungs. Fluid in the lungs, which causes shortness of breath, is called pulmonary oedema. It is a very serious condition, and can be life-threatening.

Occasionally, people with kidney failure suddenly develop pulmonary oedema, without going through the 'warning stages' of ankle and leg swelling. This can happen if they drink a lot of fluid very quickly. When pulmonary oedema comes on this quickly, it needs urgent treatment – i.e., now.

Fluid overload tends to occur mainly in kidney patients on dialysis. However, it can also be a problem for pre-dialysis patients and also for people who have had a kidney transplant.

How is fluid overload treated?

Remember, 'what goes in, has to come out'. Therefore the first treatment of fluid overload for all people with kidney failure is simply to drink less. However, this is not usually enough. Additional treatments depend on whether or not a patient is on dialysis.

1. In patients not on dialysis. If patients are pre-dialysis, or if they have a failing transplant, they will usually be given tablets called diuretics or 'water tablets' to treat fluid overload. These patients are usually able to pass urine, and the tablets work by increasing the amount of urine that is passed every day. A combination of passing more urine and drinking less usually does the trick. Two commonly used diuretic drugs are *frusemide* and *bumetanide*. Stronger diuretics, such as *mefruside* and *metolazone*, may be given as well.

If taking diuretics and drinking less does not get rid of all the fluid, it may be necessary to have some dialysis. This may be for just a few days. However, sometimes the difficulty in getting rid of fluid is a sign that kidney failure is well advanced and that dialysis may need to be permanent.

2. In patients on dialysis. Dialysis patients with fluid overload should also drink less. However, because people on dialysis usually pass little urine, diuretics don't normally work for them. A different treatment for fluid overload is needed. These patients need a combination of drinking less (usually a daily limit of 1 litre for haemodialysis patients and 1.5 litres for PD patients), and removing more water by dialysis.

Dehydration

Dehydration is the opposite of fluid overload. It occurs when there is too little water in the body. Dehydration may occur if someone does not drink enough, or if they lose fluid as a result of sweating, diarrhoea or vomiting.

It can be difficult for people to judge when they are dehydrated. However, dehydration is almost always accompanied by low blood pressure. This is easier to identify than high blood pressure. Low blood pressure makes people feel weak and dizzy when they stand up.

How is dehydration treated?

Any patient with kidney failure who is suffering from dehydration needs to drink more.

If a patient (pre-dialysis or with a failing transplant) takes diuretics, these should be reduced or stopped. If the dehydration is severe, admission to hospital for intravenous fluids (via a drip) may be necessary.

For dialysis patients, a reduction in the amount of water removed by dialysis may be needed. If haemodialysis patients are severely dehydrated, they can be given a lot of intravenous fluid during a dialysis session.

Key facts

1. Fluid balance is the balance between water coming into the body, from drinking and food, and water leaving the body, mainly in the urine or by dialysis.
2. Too much water in the body is called fluid overload. This may cause swelling of the ankles.
3. The treatment of fluid overload is to drink less, and to remove more fluid from the body. This is done by taking diuretics (water tablets), or by increasing the amount of water removed by dialysis.
4. If fluid overload is not treated, shortness of breath due to fluid in the lungs may develop. This condition – known as pulmonary oedema – needs urgent treatment at the hospital.
5. When there is too little water in the body (dehydration), dizziness may occur.
6. The treatment of dehydration is to drink more, and to remove less water from the body. This is done either by stopping diuretics, or by reducing the amount of water removed by dialysis.

4 Blood Pressure

This chapter looks at the link between blood pressure and kidney failure. It also explains the importance of blood pressure control and how this is achieved.

Introduction

The control of blood pressure is one of the important 'extra' functions performed by the kidneys. The term blood pressure means the pressure of the blood on the artery walls. This pressure goes up and down as the heart continuously squeezes and relaxes to pump blood around the body. Although the kidneys are known to help control the blood pressure, exactly how they do this is far from understood.

High blood pressure and kidney failure

High blood pressure is very common in people with kidney failure. The connection between these two conditions is two-way. High blood pressure causes kidney failure, and kidney failure causes high blood pressure. It is often difficult to know for certain whether a patient's high blood pressure has caused their kidney failure, or whether their kidney failure has caused their high blood pressure.

High blood pressure can occur in kidney patients who are pre-dialysis, who are on dialysis, or who have had a transplant. Many patients with kidney failure are taking one, two or even three types of blood pressure tablet.

Low blood pressure and kidney failure

Some people with kidney failure have a different blood pressure problem. Their blood pressure is lower than it should be. Low blood pressure is less serious than high blood pressure but it also needs to be treated.

Circulation of the blood

The main function of the blood (and the blood vessels through which it flows) is to carry things around the body. Blood carries 'good things' to parts of the body where they are needed, and also removes 'bad things' so that they can be got rid of, mainly by the kidneys in the urine.

Adults have about 10 pints of blood travelling around their body all the time. The heart acts as a pump to drive the blood through the blood vessels. There are two main types of blood vessels: arteries and veins. The arteries take blood that is rich in oxygen from the heart to all parts of the body. This oxygen provides the different parts of the body with the energy they need to do their work. The veins then take the blood (now with most of its oxygen used up) back to the heart. From there, the blood goes to the lungs to get more oxygen. It then goes back to the heart, and so the process goes on (see *diagram* next page).

Circulation of blood in the human body

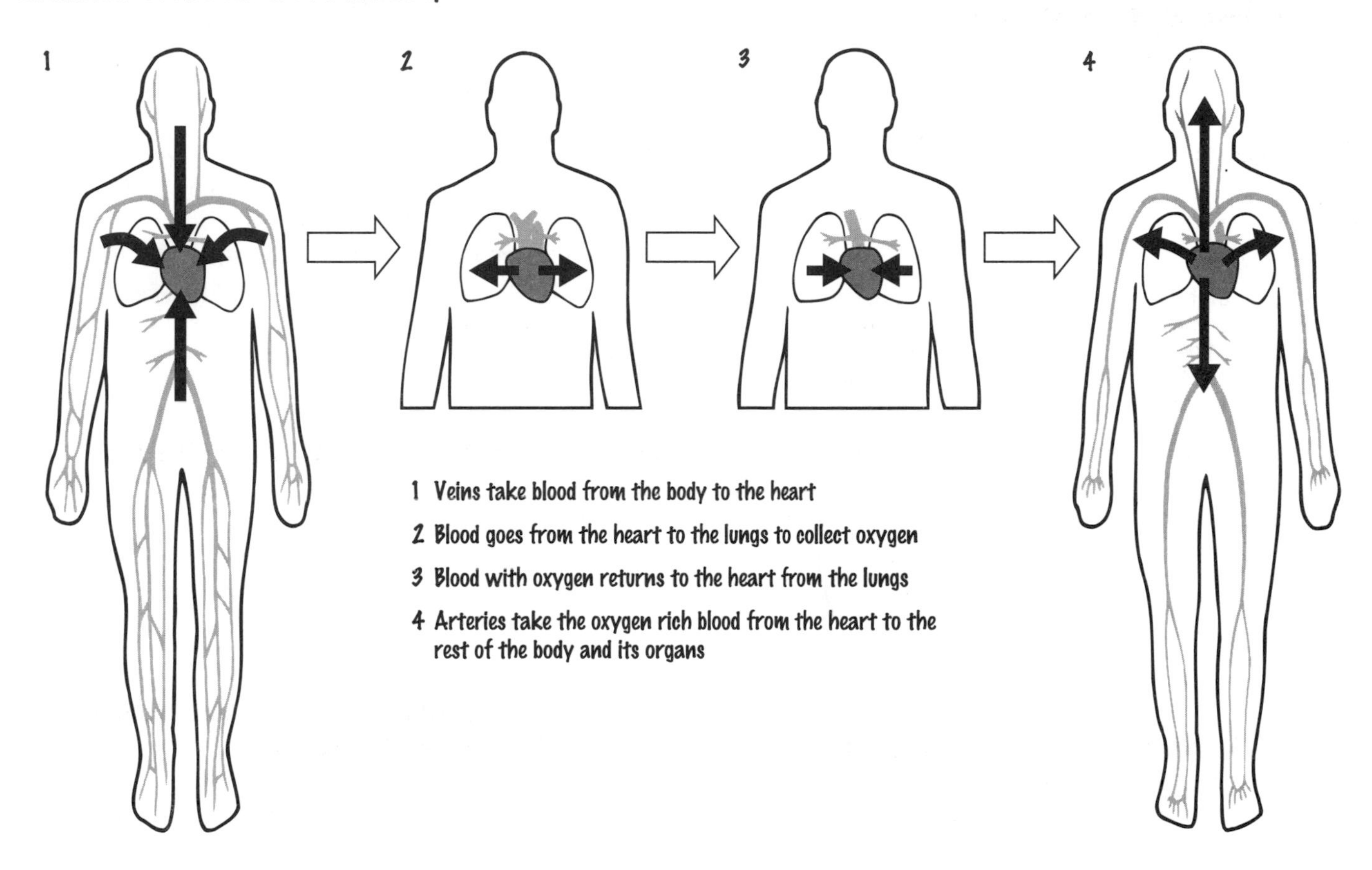

MEASURING BLOOD PRESSURE

The blood pressure is measured using a using a piece of equipment known as a sphygmomanometer (or sphyg, pronounced 'sfig'). There are various different types of sphygmomanometer, but all of them measure blood pressure in units of millimetres of mercury (mmHg).

Two readings are taken. The first reading shows the pressure of the blood when the heart squeezes, and is called the systolic blood pressure. The second reading is the pressure of the blood when the heart is relaxed. This is called the diastolic blood pressure.

The systolic pressure is always higher than the diastolic pressure, and is always recorded first. So, for example, a blood pressure of 140/80 mmHg (known as '140 over 80') means that the systolic pressure is 140 and the diastolic pressure is 80.

A reading of 140 mmHg means that the blood pressure has raised the top of the mercury (Hg) column inside the sphygmomanometer to a height of 140 millimetres.

Blood pressure

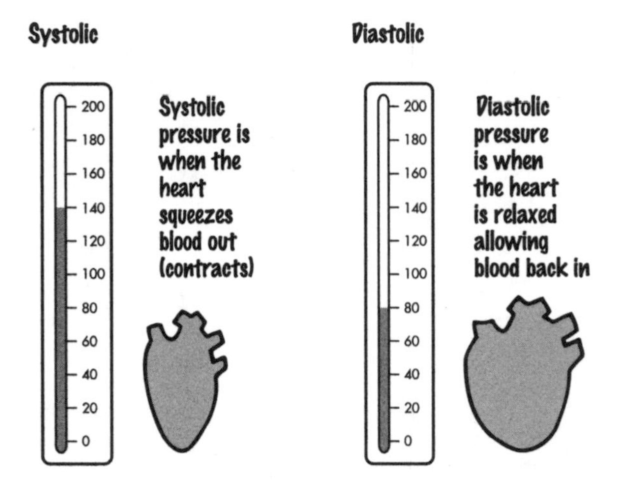

The blood pressure varies continuously throughout the heart's pumping cycle. This means that during each cycle, the systolic blood pressure is, say, 140 or 180 for only a fraction of a second.

Blood pressure also varies according to the time of day – tending to be higher in the morning and again in the early evening. There is also a difference from one arm to the other. Slight variations may also result from using different sphygmomanometers, or from how different people use the same piece of equipment.

WHAT IS 'NORMAL' BLOOD PRESSURE?

There is no such thing as normal blood pressure. Both the systolic and the diastolic blood pressure go up naturally as people get older. So, there is only a normal range of blood pressure for your age. Most doctors accept the following values as the normal range for different age groups:

AGE GROUP	BLOOD PRESSURE (in mmHg)	
	SYSTOLIC	DIASTOLIC
Under 30 years	100-120	60-70
30-60 years	110-130	70-80
Over 60 years	120-140	80-90

DOES ANXIETY AFFECT BLOOD PRESSURE?

Anxiety is definitely not a major factor in high blood pressure. Although anxiety can put the blood pressure up a little, it is a mistake to blame repeated high blood pressure readings on, for example, the 'stress of the journey' or a 'fear of seeing the doctor'.

HOW DO YOU KNOW THAT YOUR BLOOD PRESSURE IS HIGH OR LOW?

You don't. Some people with very high blood pressure suffer from headaches. But the fact that you do not have headaches does not mean that you do not have high blood pressure. The only reliable way of finding out your blood pressure is to have it measured.

If your blood pressure is very low, you may feel weak or dizzy, especially when you stand up. But there are many other causes of weakness and dizziness. So, as with high blood pressure, you cannot rely on your body to tell you that your blood pressure is low. You have to have your blood pressure checked.

WHY TREAT HIGH BLOOD PRESSURE?

There are several important reasons to treat high blood pressure. However, there is little point in treating someone for high blood pressure unless the related problems of high fat levels in the blood, being overweight and smoking are also addressed. All of these factors worsen the effects of high blood pressure.

High blood pressure increases the likelihood of a stroke or a heart attack by damaging the blood vessels. There are also 'kidney' reasons to treat high blood pressure. If blood pressure is high for a period of time, a patient with kidney failure may have to start dialysis sooner than would otherwise be necessary. This is because uncontrolled high blood pressure can accelerate kidney failure.

In fact, controlling blood pressure is the only thing proven to delay the need for dialysis in all kidney patients, whatever the cause of their kidney failure. Good blood pressure control does not mean they will never need dialysis, but it may mean that dialysis does not need to be started so soon.

WHAT DETERMINES BLOOD PRESSURE LEVELS?

A person's blood pressure is affected by the following two important factors:

1. The amount of water in the body. If there is too much water in the body (fluid overload), blood pressure will go up. If there is too little water in the body (dehydration), the blood pressure will go down. (Both fluid overload and dehydration, and their treatments, are described in *Chapter 3*.)

2. The width of the arteries. The arteries are constantly changing in width as blood flows through them. The narrower the arteries, the higher is the blood pressure.

HOW IS HIGH BLOOD PRESSURE TREATED?

There are three different ways of treating high blood pressure:

1. Reduce the amount of water in the body. If someone has fluid overload, their blood pressure will increase. This is because their blood contains more water than normal, which increases the pressure on the blood vessels. Correcting fluid overload (see *Chapter 3*), will reduce the blood pressure.

2. Vasodilator drugs. Blood pressure tablets called vasodilators lower the blood pressure by causing the arteries to widen. There are several different types of vasodilator drug:

- ACE inhibitors (e.g., *captopril, enalapril, ramipril* and *lisinopril*);
- alpha-blockers (e.g., *prazosin, doxazosin* and *terazosin*); and
- calcium antagonists (e.g., *amlodipine, nifedipine* and *diltiazem*)
- angiotensin II antagonists (e.g., *losartan, irbesartan*).

3. Beta-blocker drugs. These tablets reduce the heart rate (the number of heart beats per minute). They also lower the blood pressure, although it is not clear how they do this. Commonly used examples of beta-blockers are *atenolol, metoprolol* and *propranolol*.

ARE THE BLOOD PRESSURE TABLETS WORKING?

As blood pressure has to be very high before it causes symptoms (such as headaches), most people cannot 'feel' that their blood pressure is raised. Not surprisingly, therefore, they also cannot tell whether or not their blood pressure tablets are working. The only reliable way of knowing a person's blood pressure, and discovering whether it is responding to tablets, is for the blood pressure to be measured.

Does salt in food affect blood pressure?

Too much sodium (salt) in the body can increase the blood pressure. However, there are usually other more important factors involved (see *above*). Simply reducing the amount of salt in the diet is unlikely on its own to have much effect.

What about low blood pressure?

Low blood pressure is not as common as high blood pressure. It is normally less serious and easier to treat. This is partly because people can often feel that their blood pressure is low. So, they can also feel when it is back to normal.

Low blood pressure in people with kidney failure is usually due either to dehydration, or to taking too many blood pressure tablets. Therefore the treatment is either to drink more to correct the dehydration, or to alter the dose of blood pressure tablets.

Key facts

1. High blood pressure is very common in people with kidney failure.
2. Kidney failure causes high blood pressure, and high blood pressure causes kidney failure.
3. High blood pressure also increases the likelihood of a stroke or a heart attack.
4. You cannot reliably 'feel' your own blood pressure, especially when it is high. You have to have it checked.
5. High blood pressure can be controlled by removing fluid from your body and by taking blood pressure tablets.

5 ANAEMIA AND ERYTHROPOIETIN

This chapter explains what anaemia is, what causes it, and how the drug erythropoietin (EPO) has revolutionised the treatment.

INTRODUCTION

Many patients with kidney failure have a condition called anaemia. This means that they have a lack of red blood cells (the tiny building blocks of the body) in their body. Blood cells are produced in the bone marrow, the 'runny' bit in the middle of some bones. An important 'extra' function of the kidneys is to help control the manufacture of red blood cells in the bone marrow.

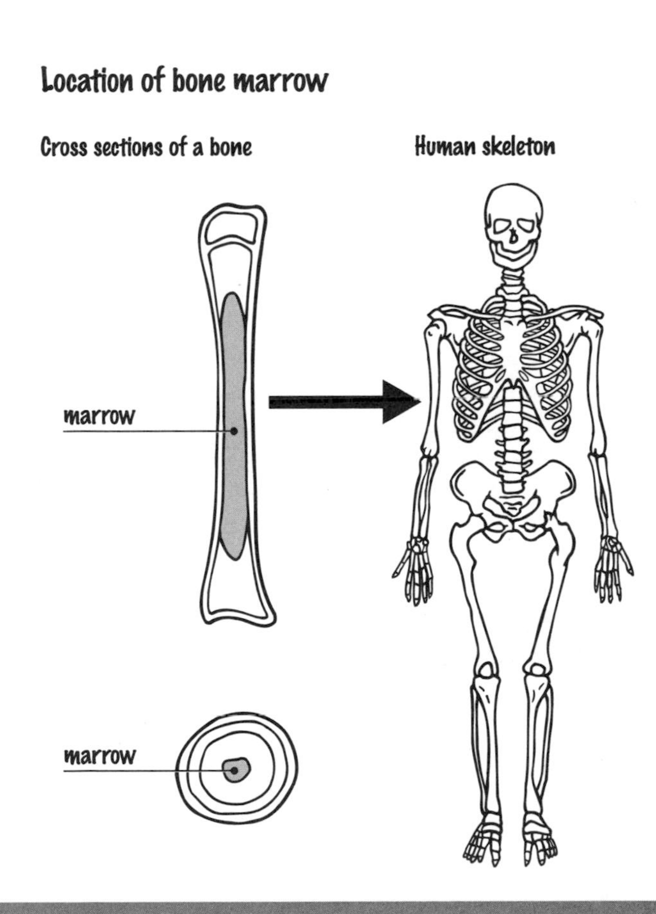

WHAT IS ANAEMIA?

Anaemia is the term for a lack of red blood cells in the body. The main symptoms are tiredness, shortness of breath, pale skin, poor appetite, irritability and low sex drive. Anaemia is probably the most important complication of kidney failure. It is the main reason why dialysis patients feel weak and tired. In fact, many of the symptoms of kidney failure are not caused by kidney failure but are actually due to anaemia.

Red blood cells are needed to carry oxygen around the body. Oxygen enters the lungs when we breathe in. From the lungs, oxygen is taken around the body in the blood. Each red blood cell contains a substance called haemoglobin. It is the haemoglobin that carries oxygen around the body. Oxygen combines with the nutrients taken in from food to provide energy to do things.

Measuring the level of haemoglobin (or 'Hb') in the blood provides a guide to the number of red cells in the blood. Normal Hb levels are 11.5-15.5 g/dl (grams per decilitre) for women, and 13-16.5 g/dl for men. If a woman's haemoglobin is below 11.5, or a man's is below 13.5 they are said to have anaemia, or to be anaemic.

Composition of the blood

Blood is made up of two parts: a liquid part and a more solid part. The liquid part is called plasma. It accounts for about 60% of the blood's volume, and is mainly water. The amount of water in the plasma is increased in fluid overload and decreased in dehydration. (Both these conditions are described in *Chapter 3*.)

The other 40% of the blood is made up of blood cells, which are so tiny that they can only be seen through a microscope. There are various different types of cells: red cells (which carry oxygen around the body), white cells (which fight infection) and platelets (involved in blood clotting). Most of the blood cells are red cells. It is these cells that give the blood its red colour. Each one looks rather like a tiny doughnut. Red cells are smaller than white cells, and larger than platelets. You have about 5 million red cells in one drop of blood.

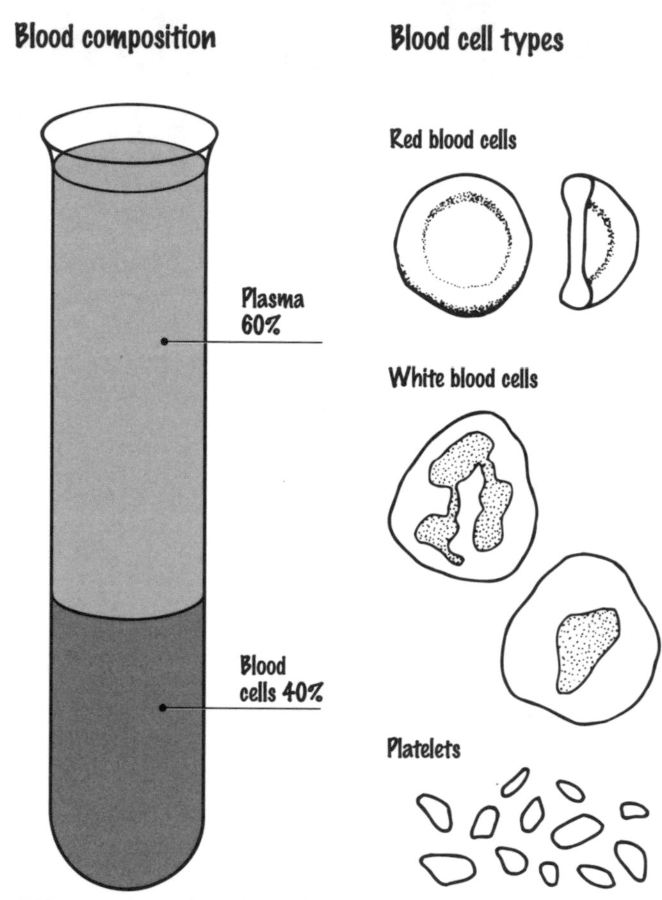

Why do people with kidney failure develop anaemia?

The main reason that kidney patients develop anaemia is simple. One of the jobs that the kidneys do, in addition to their main job of making urine, is to manage the production of red blood cells in the bone marrow. To do this, the kidneys make a substance called erythropoietin (abbreviated to EPO).

EPO travels in the blood from the kidneys to the bone marrow, where it constantly reminds the bone marrow to keep producing red cells. When someone has kidney failure, the kidneys usually make less EPO than normal. So the bone marrow 'goes to sleep' and makes fewer red cells. As a result, anaemia develops, and the patient becomes weak and tired.

Some patients with kidney failure develop anaemia even though their EPO levels are normal (or even high). This probably means that their bone marrow has a problem responding to EPO, rather than that the kidneys are not making enough EPO.

Although a lack of EPO is the main cause of anaemia in people with kidney failure, other things may contribute. For example, red blood cells do not live as long as normal (120 days) in people with kidney failure, and so must be replaced more rapidly. Also, blood may be lost during haemodialysis, or through frequent blood tests.

Problems with blood transfusions

In the past – before the introduction of EPO injections (see *below*) – blood transfusions were the only treatment for anaemia in kidney patients. Many patients had to have transfusions every couple of months, since each transfusion could reduce anaemia for a fairly short time.

Blood transfusions can cause serious problems for patients on dialysis. These include fluid overload (see *Chapter 3*), and the storing of surplus iron in the liver (which can lead to liver failure). Another problem is that whenever a transfusion of blood is received, the body produces substances called antibodies. These antibodies stay in the blood for years and can cause problems if the patient is then given a transplant. The antibodies can attack (and cause the body to reject) the new kidney.

The risks of contracting hepatitis B or C or HIV (the virus that causes AIDS) from a blood transfusion are small in the UK. Even so, if someone does not need a blood transfusion, it is better not to have one.

Blood transfusions are still sometimes needed by kidney patients – for example, after severe bleeding. In general, however, treatment with EPO has turned regular blood transfusions into a thing of the past for kidney patients.

EPO – the 'wonder drug'

Synthetically produced EPO became available as an injection in the late 1980s. By the mid-1990s, 50-75% of dialysis patients were on EPO. This drug works well in most patients, and usually gets rid of the tiredness and other symptoms caused by anaemia.

EPO is generally given in the form of an injection under the skin (called a subcutaneous injection). This is needed one to three times a week. Some patients may be asked to give their own injections. The aim of the treatment is to raise the Hb level in the blood to between 10 and 12 g/dl. Without this treatment, most patients with kidney failure will have an Hb between 6 and 8 g/dl.

A patient's response to EPO depends on how much they are given.The higher or more frequent the dose, the higher the patient's blood haemoglobin level will go. However, there is no point in making the Hb go above 10 to 12 g/dl – the patient will feel no better. In fact, problems may occur if the Hb goes over 14 g/dl. So, patients should only take EPO as prescribed.

Who needs EPO?

Patients who are on dialysis – either peritoneal dialysis (see *Chapter 8*) or haemodialysis (see *Chapter 9*) – very often need EPO. However, some doctors prefer to delay starting treatment with EPO until three months after the start of dialysis. This is because the start of dialysis will sometimes 'cure' a patient's anaemia – perhaps because dialysis removes toxins that may interfere with how the bone marrow works.

Despite this, anaemia begins long before someone needs to start dialysis. Therefore some doctors now give EPO before the start of dialysis. EPO may also be given if a transplant is failing, as anaemia often returns at this time.

Treatment with EPO has been found to be very useful even in those kidney failure patients who do not have reduced EPO levels. It is not known why giving very high doses of EPO to these patients should make such a difference to their anaemia, but it does.

Some patients with kidney failure – especially those with polycystic kidney disease (see *page 5*) – do not become anaemic, as their kidneys continue to produce EPO, even when on dialysis. They therefore do not usually need EPO treatment.

ARE THERE ANY SIDE EFFECTS?

The only common side effect of EPO is worsening of high blood pressure. This is most likely in patients who have had severe high blood pressure in the past, or in patients who are on more than one type of blood pressure tablet. If the blood pressure does increase, more blood pressure tablets may need to be taken. A combination of EPO and high blood pressure can sometimes cause fits, but this problem can usually be prevented by treating the high blood pressure.

POOR RESPONSE TO EPO TREATMENT

Most, but not all, patients respond to regular treatment with EPO. However, EPO may not work if other conditions are present. These include infections – especially repeated peritonitis in PD patients, and dialysis catheter infections in haemodialysis patients. It also may not work if there is under-dialysis (failure of dialysis to achieve target creatinine and urea levels), renal bone disease (see *Chapter 6*) or iron deficiency.

Iron deficiency is the most common reason for EPO not to work. EPO causes the body's iron stores to be used up more quickly than usual. In an attempt to spot the onset of iron deficiency, patients are given regular blood tests to measure ferritin (see *Chapter 11, page 78*). Blood ferritin levels provide a guide to the amount of iron stored in the body.

Iron deficiency can sometimes be treated with iron tablets (usually a type called ferrous sulphate). Other patients need regular iron injections. These days iron injections rather than tablets are usually given.

If EPO stops working – whatever the reason – the Hb will return to the 'normal' low level in people with kidney failure (usually 6-8 g/dl). The symptoms of anaemia will then return.

ANAEMIA AND TRANSPLANTATION

After a kidney transplant, the new kidney will start making EPO for the patient and the problem of anaemia usually goes away. Injections of EPO will then no longer be needed. However, if the transplanted kidney ever fails, anaemia will usually return, and EPO injections may be needed again.

KEY FACTS

1. Many dialysis patients have a condition called anaemia.
2. Anaemia is the major reason why dialysis patients are weak and tired.
3. The severity of anaemia is measured by a blood test called a haemoglobin (or 'Hb').
4. The lower the Hb level, the more anaemic and tired the patient will be.
5. Anaemia is easy to treat with injections of a substance called erythropoietin (EPO).
6. Patients on EPO treatment may need additional iron, either in the form of tablets or injections.

6 RENAL BONE DISEASE

This chapter provides information on the causes, prevention and treatment of renal bone disease (also known as osteodystrophy), which is a common complication of kidney failure.

INTRODUCTION

Most people with kidney failure have some degree of renal bone disease. This is because one of the 'extra' functions of the kidneys is to help make the bones strong and healthy. For the bones to be strong, the kidneys must be able to maintain a healthy balance of various substances – including calcium, phosphate and vitamin D – in the body. Kidney failure results in abnormal levels of these substances, and so leads to renal bone disease.

DEVELOPMENT OF RENAL BONE DISEASE

Blood tests will reveal abnormal levels of calcium, phosphate and vitamin D in a patient's blood very early in kidney failure, long before dialysis is required. The calcium and vitamin D levels will be too low, while the phosphate level will be too high.

Abnormalities in calcium, phosphate and vitamin D levels do not usually lead to problems that a patient is likely to notice until after the start of dialysis. However, treatment should be started at an early stage to prevent weakening of the bones.

Without treatment, renal bone disease can lead to pain in the bones, especially in the back, hips, legs and knees. The weakened bones also become increasingly prone to fracture. However, early recognition and treatment of renal bone disease means that bone pain and fractures are now uncommon in kidney patients.

WHAT CAUSES RENAL BONE DISEASE?

There are three main causes of renal bone disease:

1. Low calcium levels in the blood. Calcium is a mineral that strengthens the bones. It is obtained from some foods, especially dairy products, eggs and green vegetables. In our bodies, calcium is stored in the bones. There is also some calcium in the blood. The kidneys normally help to keep calcium in the bones. In people with kidney failure, calcium drains out of the bones and is lost from the body. This leads to a fall in the level of calcium in the blood.

The normal blood calcium level is between 2.2 and 2.6 mmol/l (millimoles per litre of blood). In kidney patients, the level of calcium in the blood may fall below 2.0 mmol/l. Treatment can keep the calcium level up quite easily.

2. High phosphate levels in the blood. Phosphate is another mineral that strengthens the bones. Foods that contain phosphate include dairy products, nuts and meat. Like calcium, phosphate is stored in the body in the bones and is also present in the blood. The kidneys normally help to keep the right amount in the blood – not too much, not too little. In people with kidney failure, phosphate builds up in the blood.

The normal level of phosphate in the blood is 0.8 to 1.4 mmol/l. In kidney patients, it is very common for the blood phosphate level to be high, rising to more than 2.0 mmol/l. Unfortunately, it is quite difficult to keep phosphate levels normal. High phosphate levels are thought to cause itching.

3. Low vitamin D levels in the blood. Vitamin D is needed in the body so that calcium from the diet can be absorbed into the body and used to strengthen the bones. Vitamin D is found in some foods, especially margarine and butter. However, most of our vitamin D is made by the skin (a process that only occurs if the skin is stimulated by sunlight). Unfortunately, vitamin D from food and from the skin are in a form which the body cannot use directly. The kidneys are responsible for transforming vitamin D into a useable substance.

Blood levels of the useable form of vitamin D are not usually measured, as the blood test is expensive and difficult to do. If they were measured, they would be low. It is quite easy to provide additional vitamin D as tablets or injections, though not all kidney patients need it. Often, it will be enough just to control the levels of calcium and phosphate.

A combination of causes

Doctors do not know which of the three main causes of renal bone disease comes first. Nor do they know what leads to what. They do know, however, that although any one of these causes can lead to problems, a combination of the three is usually present in people with kidney failure. More importantly, each of the causes tends to have a 'knock-on' effect, worsening the other two abnormalities. For example, a high phosphate level tends to lower the calcium level, and vice versa. It is therefore important to treat all three causes (see *page 31*).

Parathyroid hormone and kidney failure

Parathyroid hormone (PTH) is a substance produced by four tiny glands called the parathyroid glands. These glands are situated in the front of the neck. When someone has kidney failure, the parathyroid glands become over-active and produce too much PTH. Raised PTH levels can aggravate renal bone disease.

Location of the parathyroid glands

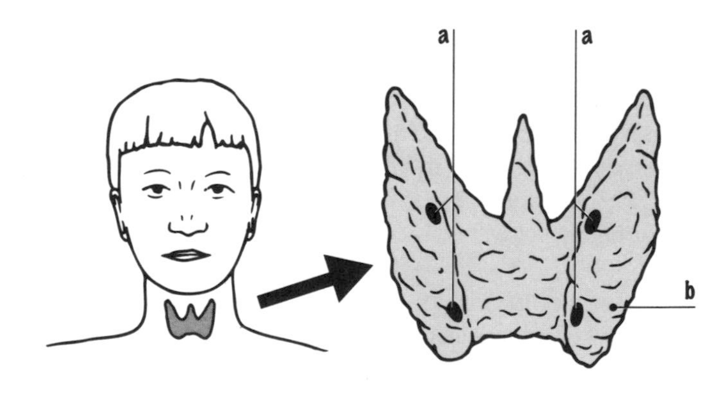

The parathyroid glands (a) are four tiny glands located at the back of the thyroid gland (b), in the neck

HOW IS RENAL BONE DISEASE MONITORED?

The levels of calcium and phosphate in a kidney patient's blood can tell us what is happening in the bones at the time of the test. However, these levels provide little information about the future.

The best guide to the progress and severity of renal bone disease is the amount of parathyroid hormone (PTH) in the blood. PTH tells us much more about the long-term health of the bones. Changes in blood PTH can tell us about what will happen to the bones in the future – the lower the PTH, the better.

Renal bone disease begins very early in kidney failure. It is therefore a good idea for doctors to measure a patient's blood PTH even before dialysis is necessary. Once dialysis has started, most doctors will measure the blood PTH every six months or so. A high level indicates a problem with the bones. Doctors will then start a range of treatments to help prevent any worsening of the problem. Even very high PTH levels can usually be lowered with the right tablets.

HOW IS RENAL BONE DISEASE TREATED?

Treatment may be needed for each of the three main causes of renal bone disease.

1. Raising low calcium levels. Patients on dialysis can obtain some extra calcium from the dialysis fluid. This happens because there is more calcium in some dialysis fluids than there is in the blood. Calcium passes from the stronger solution (the dialysis fluid) into the patient's blood (the weaker solution) by a process called diffusion. (See *Chapter 7* for more information on diffusion.)

For many kidney patients, extra calcium from dialysis is not enough They also need calcium in the form of a drug. This drug is calcium carbonate (commonly taken in a preparation called *Calcichew*). Calcium carbonate tablets may need to be taken every day to look after the long-term health of the bones.

Although the main job of calcium carbonate in kidney patients is to reduce blood phosphate levels (see *below, point 2*), calcium carbonate also has the effect of raising blood calcium levels. Blood calcium levels are also raised by treatment with vitamin D (see *below, point 3*).

Treatment is most successful when blood calcium levels are driven to the upper limit of normal. So, the target blood calcium level for someone with kidney failure should be 2.5 to 2.6 mmol/l (given the normal range of 2.2 to 2.6 mmol/l). This target applies all the time for a peritoneal dialysis (PD) patient, and before dialysis for a patient on haemodialysis.

2. Lowering high phosphate levels. Dialysis removes some phosphate from the blood, but it does not do this very efficiently. Most patients therefore need further treatment to control phosphate levels.

To lower their blood phosphate levels, kidney patients are usually given tablets called phosphate binders. Two different types of phosphate binders are calcium carbonate (see *above, point 1*) and aluminium hydroxide. Aluminium hydroxide is rarely used these days. To be effective, any type of phosphate binder needs to be taken just before food, and not together with iron tablets.

If the combination of dialysis and phosphate-binding tablets fails to control a patient's phosphate levels, then it may be necessary for the patient to have more dialysis, or to eat less high-phosphate foods (see *Chapter 12, page 82*), or both of these.

Even with treatment, a kidney patient's blood phosphate rarely returns to the normal level of 0.8 to 1.4 mmol/l. So, the target blood phosphate level is not normal. It is a level of less than 1.8 mmol/l. This target applies all the time for a PD patient, and before dialysis for a haemodialysis patient.

3. Raising low vitamin D levels. In a few patients, renal bone disease continues to be a problem even when the blood calcium and phosphate levels are brought under control. Treatment with a vitamin D preparation is then needed. The most commonly used type is called *alfacalcidol*. Vitamin D treatment works in two ways: it provides the vitamin D that is lacking and it increases blood calcium levels (see *above, point 1*). PD patients receive vitamin D in the form of a tablet. Haemodialysis patients receive it either as tablet, or as an injection given during dialysis.

PARATHYROIDECTOMY

In most patients, correcting the blood levels of calcium, phosphate and vitamin D is enough to control renal bone disease, and to cause PTH levels to fall.

In a few patients, however, this treatment plan is not sufficient, and blood PTH levels continue to rise. When this happens, the blood calcium tends to rise to above normal (it is usually low in kidney failure). At this stage, the blood phosphate is usually very high. This combination of an extremely high PTH, a high calcium and a very high phosphate level cannot be treated by dialysis and tablets alone. It is then necessary to carry out an operation to remove the parathyroid glands. This operation is called a parathyroidectomy.

If an operation is not performed, the blood vessels can become 'furred up' with calcium, which can be very dangerous. Calcium may also be deposited in the eyes (making them red and itchy) or in the skin (which can cause parts of the skin to go black and die). A parathyroidectomy is a very effective operation. It returns blood calcium levels to normal, and can prevent these complications.

A parathyroidectomy operation takes 1 to 2 hours, and requires a hospital stay of 5 to 7 days after the operation. For the next few weeks, frequent blood calcium checks will be needed. This is because blood calcium levels can fall to a very low level after the operation. It is often necessary for patients to take high doses of calcium carbonate and/or vitamin D after a parathyroidectomy. These can usually be stopped at a later date.

TRANSPLANTS AND RENAL BONE DISEASE

If a patient receives a transplant and the new kidney works well, the blood levels of calcium, phosphate, vitamin D and PTH will usually return to normal, or near normal. Renal bone disease then improves, although it never really goes away completely.

If a transplanted kidney never functions properly, or if it starts to fail after working well, renal bone disease will become a problem. It is therefore important to pay attention to the calcium, phosphate and PTH levels even after a transplant.

BONE PAIN DUE TO DIALYSIS AMYLOIDOSIS

Renal bone disease is not the only cause of bone pain in patients with kidney failure. Bone pain can also be caused by a condition called dialysis amyloidosis.

This condition seems to develop 10 years or so after the start of kidney failure. It is caused by poor removal by dialysis of a protein called amyloid. This causes a build-up of amyloid in the body, which continues even when a patient starts dialysis. After a time, amyloid is deposited in the joints all over the body, especially in the wrists and shoulders. This leads to joint and bone pain.

At present, there is no effective treatment for this condition in dialysis patients. Its progress is halted – to an extent – by transplantation.

KEY FACTS

1. Renal bone disease is an important complication of kidney failure.
2. Without treatment, renal bone disease can cause bone pain and fractures.
3. Renal bone disease starts early in kidney failure but does not usually cause problems until after dialysis has begun.
4. Renal bone disease is caused by low levels of calcium and vitamin D in the blood, and by high blood levels of phosphate.
5. A combination of dialysis and tablets usually reverses these problems.
6. The level of parathyroid hormone (PTH) in the blood is the best long-term indication of the health of the bones.
7. If dialysis and tablets fail to control renal bone disease, an operation called a parathyroidectomy may be necessary to remove the parathyroid glands in the neck.

7 DIALYSIS – THE BASICS

This chapter describes what dialysis is, and explains how it works. The points covered apply to both peritoneal dialysis and haemodialysis.

INTRODUCTION

This is the first of four chapters which explain the treatment options available to people with kidney failure. There are basically two ways of treating kidney failure: dialysis (see also *Chapters 8 and 9*) and transplantation (see *Chapter 10*). There is currently no cure.

WHAT IS DIALYSIS?

Dialysis is an artificial way of doing the work of the kidneys. It clears the waste products (of food) from the blood, and it also removes excess water. Dialysis thus performs the two main functions of the kidneys: toxin clearance (see *Chapter 2*) and maintaining fluid balance (see *Chapter 3*).

There are two different types of dialysis: peritoneal dialysis, often called PD (see *Chapter 8*), and haemodialysis (see *Chapter 9*).

HOW DOES DIALYSIS WORK?

Even though at first sight PD and haemodialysis may seem quite different, they work in similar ways:

- Waste products are cleared from the blood by a process called diffusion (see *page 35*).
- Excess water is removed from the blood by a process known as ultrafiltration (see *page 36*).
- Wastes and water pass into a special liquid – called the dialysis fluid or dialysate – for removal from the body.
- A thin layer of tissue or plastic, known as the dialysis membrane, keeps the dialysis fluid and blood apart.

THE ROLE OF THE DIALYSIS FLUID

Both of the key processes involved in dialysis – i.e., diffusion and ultrafiltration – depend on the use of a dialysis fluid. Body wastes and excess fluid can only pass from the blood if they have somewhere to go. The dialysis fluid provides the 'container' in which they are removed from the body. The dialysis solution is slightly different in each type of dialysis but it does the same job.

The chemical content of the dialysis fluid affects the flow of substances between the blood and the dialysis fluid. During dialysis, body wastes and excess fluid pass from the blood into the dialysis fluid. Other substances, such as calcium, will flow in the opposite direction, from the dialysis fluid into the blood.

THE DIALYSIS MEMBRANE

Dialysis solution is toxic to the body if it flows directly into the blood. It is therefore important to keep the dialysis fluid separate from the blood. This is done by using a dialysis membrane, which looks similar to a very thin piece of 'cling film'.

The dialysis membrane has thousands of tiny holes in it. These holes are big enough to let water, body wastes and various other substances through, yet small enough to keep the blood cells and proteins inside the blood vessels. So, the dialysis membrane acts as a 'leaky barrier' between the blood and the dialysis fluid.

In haemodialysis, the membrane used is artificial, made from a type of plastic. The membrane, folded over many thousands of times, is situated in an artificial kidney (also called a dialyser). Dialysis takes place outside the patient's body, in the artificial kidney.

In PD, a natural membrane inside the abdomen, called the peritoneum, is used. The peritoneum lines the inside wall of the abdomen and covers all the abdominal organs (the stomach, bowels, liver, etc.). It is a thin layer of tissue rather like a thin balloon in appearance and texture.

WASTE REMOVAL BY DIFFUSION

Diffusion is one of the key processes involved in dialysis. It is a process by which substances pass from a stronger to a weaker solution.

Diffusion works in the same way as a tea bag. When hot water is poured over a tea bag, the tea comes out of the bag and into the water. The surface of the teabag is like the dialysis membrane as it lets tea drain out of the tea leaves, but does not let the tea leaves out themselves. The tea mixes with the water until the tea is the same colour throughout the cup.

The process of diffusion

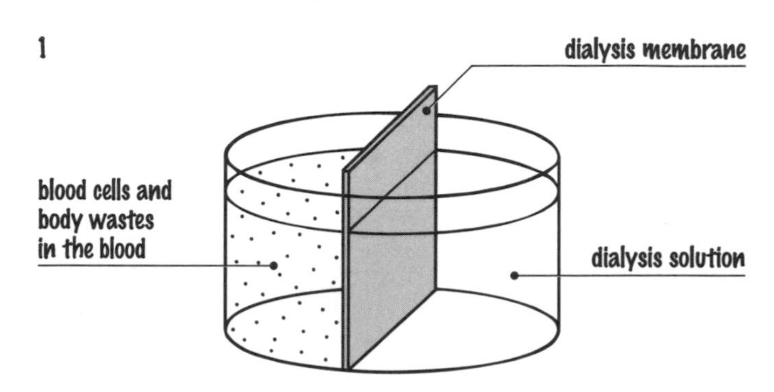

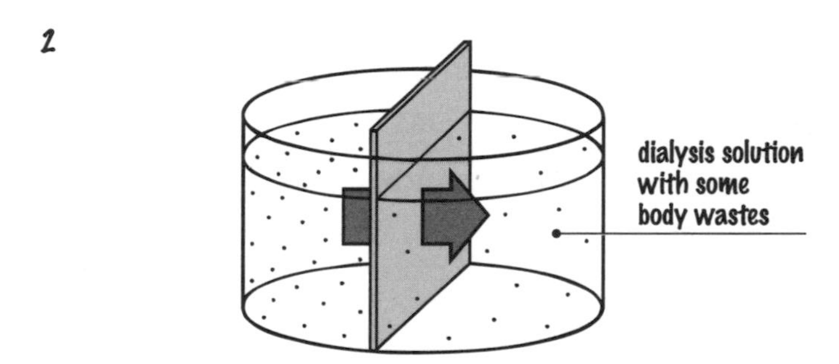

Blood cells are too big to pass through the dialysis membrane, but body wastes begin to diffuse (pass) into the dialysis solution

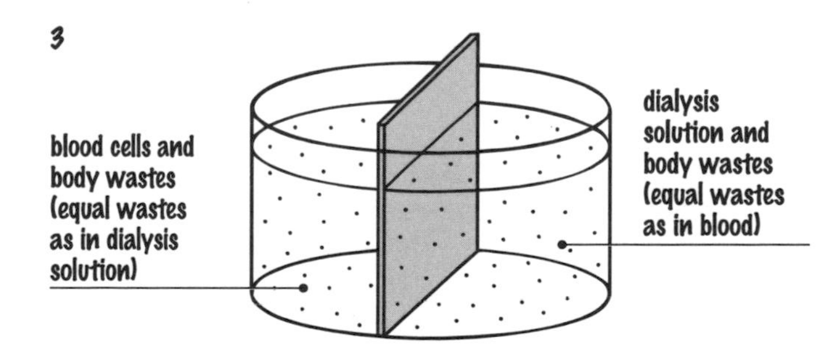

Diffusion is complete. Body wastes have diffused through the membrane, and now there are equal amounts of wastes in both the blood and the dialysis solution

People with kidney failure have a lot of body wastes in their blood. If the blood is put next to a dialysis fluid that does not have any of these wastes in it, the wastes will pass from the blood into the dialysis fluid. So, if we want to remove unwanted substances (such as urea or creatinine) from the blood, we need a dialysis fluid that contains little or none of those substances.

As dialysis proceeds, there comes a point at which there are equal amount of wastes in the blood and in the dialysis fluid (like when the tea stops changing colour). The process of diffusion then stops, and no more wastes will move across. This is the basic principle underlying dialysis.

Diffusion also works the 'other way'. If the amount of a substance is higher in the dialysis fluid than in the blood, then that substance will pass from the dialysis fluid into the blood. So, if we want to add useful substances (such as calcium) to the body via the blood, we use dialysis fluid that contains a lot of those substances.

FLUID REMOVAL BY ULTRAFILTRATION

Ultrafiltration – the other key process involved in dialysis – occurs at the same time as diffusion. It is the process by which excess fluid (mainly water) is drawn out of the blood during dialysis. Ultrafiltration happens in slightly different ways in haemodialysis and PD.

In haemodialysis, the water is 'sucked' from the blood by the kidney machine. The amount of water to be removed during a session of haemodialysis can be varied, from a lot to a little, depending on how the machine is set up.

In PD, a substance is put into the dialysis fluid which 'sucks' the water from the blood. The most commonly used substance is glucose (i.e., sugar). The way the

The process of ultrafiltration in PD

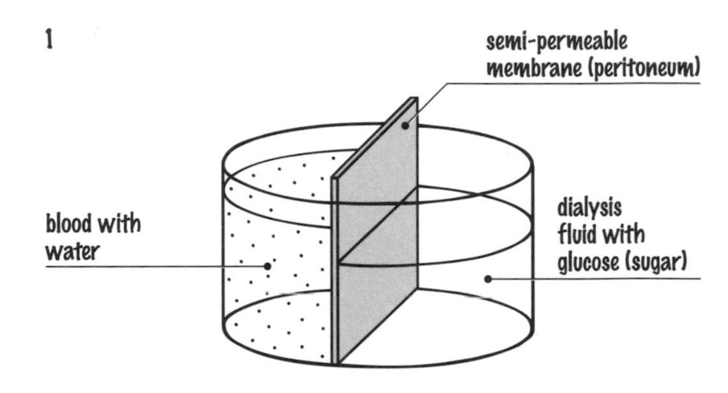

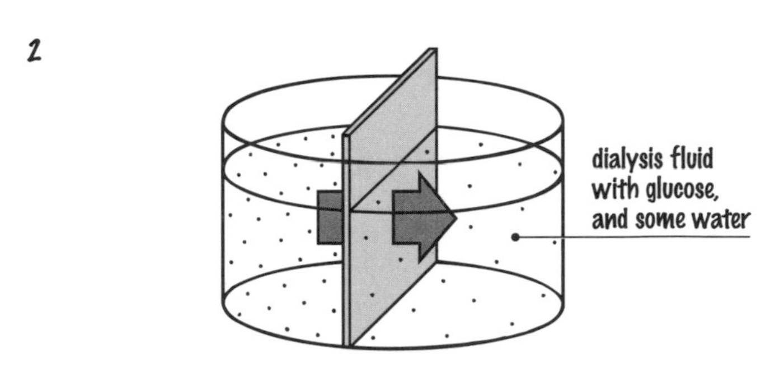

Blood cells are too big to pass through the semi-permeable membrane, but water in the blood is drawn into the dialysis fluid by the glucose

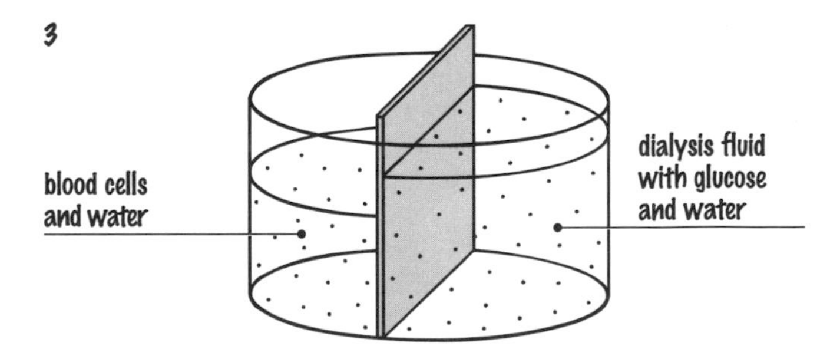

Ultrafiltration is complete. Water has been drawn through the peritoneum by the glucose in the dialysis fluid. There is now extra water in the dialysis fluid which needs to be changed

glucose sucks water from the blood is the same way as a tree draws water up from the ground to its highest leaves. It depends on a process called osmosis.

Osmosis occurs when a liquid from a weak solution (e.g., water in the blood) passes through a semi-permeable membrane (e.g., the dialysis membrane) into a stronger solution (e.g., of glucose in the dialysis fluid). By this means, water is lost from the blood, and the glucose solution is diluted.

The amount of water drawn from the blood depends on the amount of sugar in the solution – the more sugar, the more water will be removed. Hence in PD, there are different strengths of dialysis bag – with 'strong' bags containing more sugar than 'weak' bags. The choice of bag depends on how much water needs to be removed from the patient's blood: a strong bag will remove more water than a weak bag.

PD OR HAEMODIALYSIS?

Both methods of dialysis are equally effective. Haemodialysis works much more quickly than PD and so only has to be done in short sessions (taking 3 to 5 hours), usually three times a week. PD is a much gentler form of dialysis and so needs to be performed every day.

In the UK, approximately half of the patients on dialysis are treated by haemodialysis, and the other half by PD. In fact, it is possible for most patients to have either type of treatment. Indeed, most patients will experience both during their life with kidney failure.

In most other developed countries, PD is not quite so common. For example, only about 20% of patients in the USA are treated by PD. There are various theories as to why this is the case.

It could be that doctors in the USA do not believe that PD is as effective as haemodialysis. Or it could be that patients in the USA prefer to be looked after in hospital renal units, rather than having the responsibility of looking after themselves at home.

It could also be due to the fact that doctors in some countries are paid according to how many patients they treat by the different types of dialysis. Doctors in these countries often receive more money for haemodialysis patients than they do for patients on PD.

KEY FACTS

1. Dialysis is the word used to describe the removal of body wastes and water from the blood.
2. There are two types of dialysis: haemodialysis and peritoneal dialysis. Both work in a similar way.
3. There are two main processes involved in dialysis: diffusion and ultrafiltration. Diffusion removes the body wastes and ultrafiltration removes the excess water.
4. In the UK, approximately half of the patients on dialysis have PD and the other half have haemodialysis.
5. Most patients can have either type of dialysis.

8 Peritoneal Dialysis

This chapter concentrates on peritoneal dialysis (PD), the newer of the two types of dialysis that may be used to treat people with kidney failure.

Introduction

Peritoneal dialysis (PD) is one of the two types of dialysis that may be used to treat people with kidney failure. In PD, the process of dialysis (see *Chapter 7*) takes place inside the patient's body, using the peritoneum (the natural lining of the abdomen) as the dialysis membrane. PD has been available in the UK since the late 1970s. It has proved to be a highly successful alternative to the 'traditional' form of dialysis known as haemodialysis (see *Chapter 9*).

Who can be treated by PD?

PD is a suitable treatment for most people with end-stage renal failure (ESRF). However, there are a few exceptions:

- People who have had several major abdominal operations may not be able to have PD. This is because a scarred peritoneum may not be an effective dialysis membrane.

- PD requires a lot of commitment from kidney patients and their families. Kidney patients on PD are responsible for exchanging their own dialysis fluid (see *page 41*). They perform these exchanges in their own homes. For this reason, PD is not recommended if patients are unable to care for themselves and do not have someone available full-time to help them with their exchanges.

What does PD do?

PD (like haemodialysis) takes over some of the work that is normally done by the kidneys. It removes the waste products of food (toxin clearance, see *Chapter 2*) and it removes excess water from the body (see *Chapter 3*). It can also be used to give people various substances that they are lacking, such as calcium or bicarbonate.

PD and haemodialysis are equivalent techniques in terms of the amount of dialysis they can deliver (about 5% of the function of two normal kidneys). Both relieve the symptoms of kidney failure and both enable patients to go back to work.

How does PD work?

The basic principles of dialysis are the same for PD and haemodialysis. (These principles are explained in detail in *Chapter 7*.) Briefly, both types of dialysis use a special liquid (called the dialysis fluid, dialysis solution or dialysate) and a membrane (called the dialysis membrane) to do some of the work of the kidneys. In PD, the dialysis membrane is the patient's own peritoneum (see *below*).

The dialysis fluid provides the 'container' in which waste products and excess water can be removed from the body. The dialysis membrane acts as a filter. It keeps the dialysis fluid and the blood separate from each other, but it allows certain substances and water to pass through it. During dialysis, substances pass from the blood into the dialysis fluid (and vice versa). They do this by a process called diffusion, by which substances pass from a stronger to a weaker solution (see *page 35*). At the same time, ultrafiltration occurs (see *page 36*). Excess water passes from the blood into the dialysis fluid by a process called osmosis, in which liquid in a weaker solution passes into a stronger one.

THE PERITONEUM

The essential difference between PD and haemodialysis is that in PD, the dialysis process takes place inside the patient's abdomen, using a natural membrane – the peritoneum – as the dialysis membrane. It is from the peritoneum that PD (peritoneal dialysis) gets its name.

The peritoneum is a natural membrane that lines the inside of the abdominal wall and covers all the abdominal organs (the stomach, bowels, liver, etc.). It resembles a balloon in appearance and texture but has lots of extremely tiny holes in it. These holes allow the peritoneum to be used as a dialysis membrane. As blood flows through the blood vessels in the peritoneum, it flows past the holes. Although the holes are extremely tiny, water and toxins can easily pass through, but blood cells are too large. In this way, the peritoneum in PD works as a 'natural filter', performing the same function as the 'artificial filter' used in haemodialysis.

The peritoneum has two layers – one lining the inside of the abdominal wall, the other lining the abdominal organs. Between these two layers is a space. This space is called the peritoneal cavity. During PD, it is the peritoneal cavity that is used as a reservoir for the dialysis fluid. Normally, the peritoneal cavity contains only about 100 ml of liquid. In fact, it can expand to hold up to 5 litres of liquid. (Women who have been pregnant can vouch for this.)

The position of the peritoneal cavity

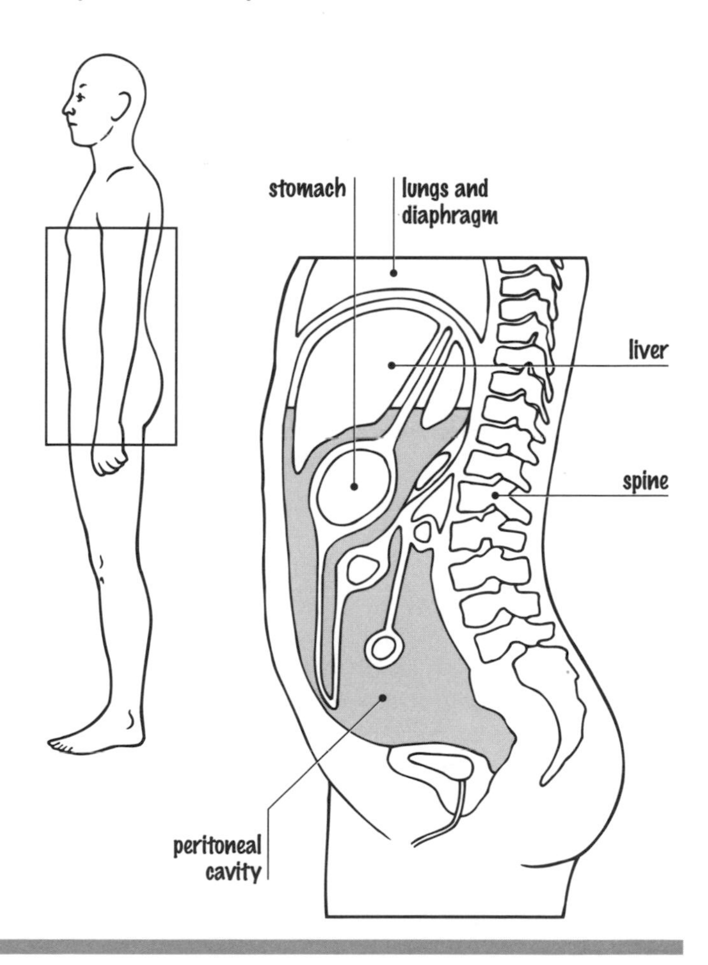

HOW IS PD DONE?

PD needs to be done every day. It consists of the following three stages:

1. The peritoneal cavity is filled with 1.5 to 3 litres of dialysis fluid from a dialysis bag. (The amount varies, depending on a patient's individual needs and the type of dialysis fluid used.)

2. The dialysis fluid is left inside the peritoneum to allow dialysis to take place. (The length of time it is left there varies, from between 30 minutes to 8 hours, depending on individual requirements and the type of PD.)

3. The 'used' fluid, containing the water and toxins that the kidneys would normally have passed into the urine, is drained out of the body and discarded, usually down the toilet.

OPERATION TO INSERT A PD CATHETER

To receive PD, a kidney patient first needs to have a small operation. During the operation (which is performed using a local or a general anaesthetic), a plastic tube is permanently inserted into the abdomen (see *diagram*). This tube is called a PD catheter. It is about 30 cm (12 in) long and as wide as a pencil.

The PD catheter is placed through the lower abdominal wall, into the peritoneal cavity. Half of the catheter lies inside the abdomen, and half lies outside. It comes out on the right or the left, under the navel (tummy button). The PD catheter acts as a permanent pathway into the peritoneal cavity from the outside world. It is the PD patient's dialysis 'lifeline'.

Patients are usually allowed to go home 1 or 2 days after the operation. The catheter is 'left alone' for 5 days or more after the operation before it can be used for dialysis. This allows it to 'settle in' and gives the abdominal wound time to heal.

PD catheter – position inside the body

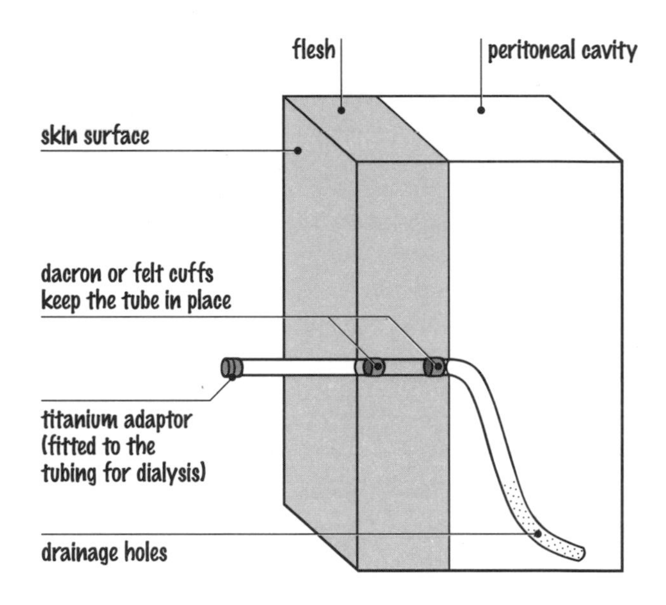

THE TRAINING

PD is performed by patients themselves, in their own homes. They therefore need proper training to perform their own dialysis fluid exchanges. This training is usually given to patients a week or so after their PD catheter operation.

Before anyone is expected to carry out their own dialysis, they will be trained in all aspects of their care by specialist nurses. Most patients can become competent in the exchange technique in 3 to 14 days. Some hospitals train patients as an in-patient, some as an out-patient. When patients first go home and have to do the exchanges by themselves, they may find it a bit daunting. However, within a few weeks most patients find that they are doing the dialysis by themselves with no problems.

METHODS OF FLUID EXCHANGE

The way that the dialysis fluid is exchanged depends on the type of PD.

There are two main types of PD, which differ only in the way that the dialysis fluid is exchanged. The two different types of PD are:

1. Continuous ambulatory peritoneal dialysis (CAPD). 'Continuous' means 'all the time' and ambulatory' means 'while you walk around'. In this form of PD, patients walk around with the dialysis fluid in their abdomen. At the end of each period of dialysis, they have to change the dialysis fluid themselves (see *diagrams, below* and *page 42* for details).

2. Automated peritoneal dialysis (APD). 'Automated' means that a machine changes the dialysis fluid for the patient. The patient remains connected to the machine while dialysis is taking place, usually at night (see *page 42* for details).

Fluid exchanges in CAPD

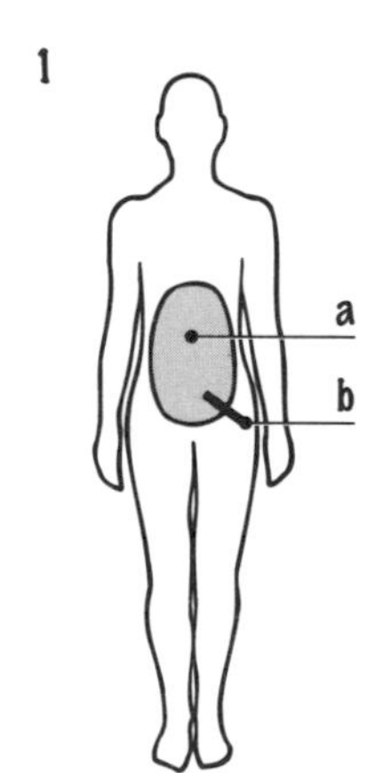

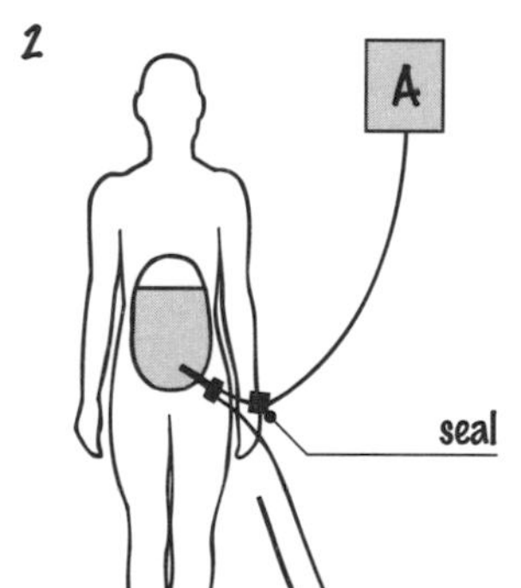

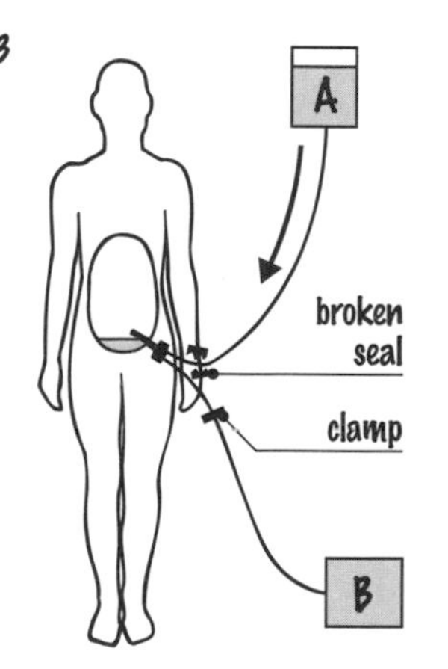

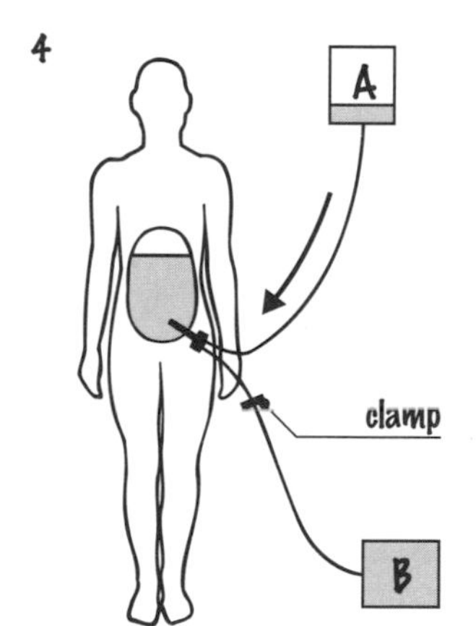

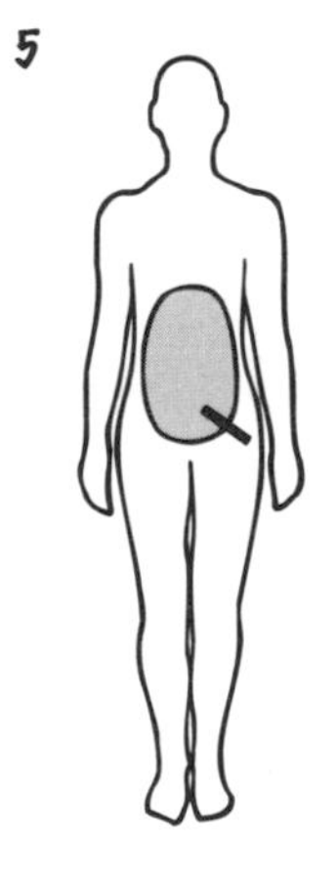

a peritoneal cavity
b catheter tube

1 Patient with used dialysis fluid ready to exchange

2 A Y-shaped tube is connected to the patient's PD catheter. At one end of the Y tubing is a bag full of fresh dialysis fluid (A). Used fluid is drained into the empty bag (B) which is at the other end of the Y tubing

3 When all the used fluid has drained into the drainage bag (B), the drainage tube is clamped to stop more fluid flowing down the tube. The seal is broken and fresh fluid is then drained into the peritoneal cavity from bag A

4 Once all the fresh fluid is inside the patient all the tubes are clamped and the bags are disconnected, leaving the patient free from the equipment until the next time a dialysis exchange is due

5 Patient with fresh dialysis fluid

FLUID EXCHANGES IN CAPD

When patients are on CAPD, they do their own fluid exchanges. They drain 1.5 to 3 litres of dialysis fluid into their abdomen, leave it there for 4 to 8 hours, and then drain it out. This is done four to five times a day – every day. It is as simple as that. With practice, an exchange of fluid can be done in about 20 minutes. Exchanges are simple to do and can be performed almost anywhere.

The dialysis fluid is kept in sealed plastic bags. The bags are connected and disconnected to the peritoneal catheter with a system of tubes and clamps. (How this is done is shown in the *diagrams* on *page 41*.)

There are no 'set' times to carry out the exchanges. However, a four bag regime 'fits' into a typical day. For example, the first bag might be exchanged before breakfast, the second before lunch, the third before the evening meal, and the fourth before going to bed (leaving the fluid for the last exchange in through the night). It is easy for patients to adapt the timing of exchanges to their own individual needs. For example, if a patient wants to go out for the day, they could delay the mid-day exchange, and do two 'quick bags' (say, 3 hours apart) after they come home.

FLUID EXCHANGES IN APD

APD uses a machine to do the dialysis fluid exchanges for the patient. The machine is usually placed in the bedroom and does the exchanges while the patient is asleep. Some APD machines are only the size of a video recorder (see *illustration*) and make it possible for patients to do exchanges in different places.

Most patients need to spend 8 to 10 hours attached to the machine every night. This enables the machine to perform an average of six exchanges of 1.5 to 3 litres of dialysis fluid each night. The length of time that PD fluid is left in the abdomen before it is exchanged by the machine varies from between about 30 minutes and 3 hours. After spending the night on the machine, most people on APD keep fluid inside their peritoneum during the daytime without needing to exchange it.

A portable APD machine

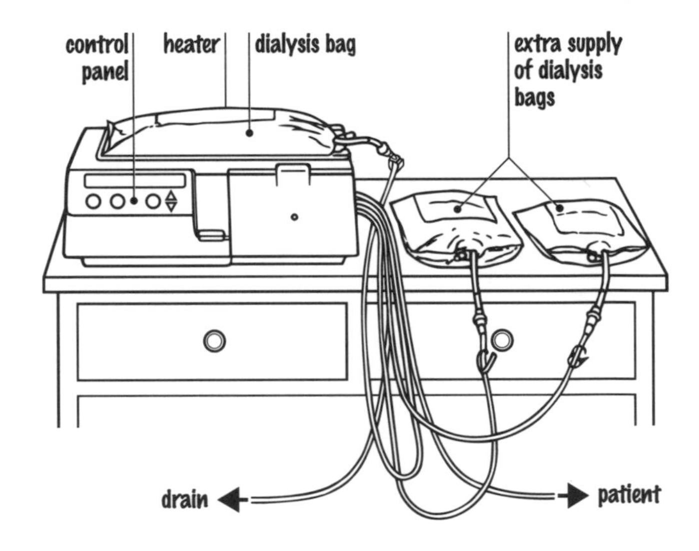

CAPD OR APD?

In most renal units in the UK, about 80% of the PD patients currently do CAPD and 20% do APD. However, the number of patients doing APD is growing all the time. Different patients may be better suited to either CAPD or APD for a number of reasons.

1. How the peritoneum works. The main medical reason why a doctor may choose either CAPD or APD for a patient relates to the way the patient's peritoneum works during dialysis.

Some patients, called 'high transporters', have a peritoneum which works best with more frequent exchanges of dialysis fluid. High transporters are usually more suited to APD, because the machine is able to do rapid exchanges of dialysis fluid whilst they sleep.

Other patients, called 'low transporters', will get more dialysis if the fluid is left inside them for longer periods. Low transporters are generally better suited to CAPD.

A test has been developed to find out whether patients are 'high' or 'low transporters'. This test is called a Peritoneal Equilibration Test, or PET, and is usually performed in hospital by a nurse. It takes 4 hours to complete and involves doing just one CAPD exchange. The test measures how quickly the toxins move out of the patient's bloodstream and into the dialysis fluid. If the toxins move quickly, the patient is called a 'high transporter'. If the toxins move slowly, the patient is a 'low transporter'.

2. Patient size. APD can also be particularly good for patients who require a lot of dialysis – for example, large people, especially those who no longer pass urine. This is because the machine can do more fluid exchanges than patients are able to do themselves with CAPD. Also, as the patients are lying down, they may be more able to tolerate bigger volumes of dialysis fluid. In these ways, APD can remove more waste toxins than CAPD. Even so, for some very large patients, APD during the night may not be enough. Such patients commonly need an additional CAPD exchange at tea-time.

3. Patients with a carer. APD is a possible treatment option for patients who need a carer to perform dialysis for them, such as the elderly, infirm or very young.

4. Employment reasons. Since APD exchanges are done during the night, this form of dialysis can be particularly suitable for patients who work or who are in full-time education.

Bigger bags and stronger bags

Whatever the type of PD (either CAPD or APD), the ability to remove toxins can be raised by increasing either the volume of fluid used, or the number of exchanges, or both. A larger bag will remove more toxins (and a little more water) than a smaller bag. The dialysis needs of patients depend partly on their body size (see *Chapter 2*). Big people usually need 'big bags' (2.5 or 3 litres of dialysis fluid).

The ability of PD fluid to remove water is affected by the amount of glucose (sugar) in the bag – the more glucose in the bag, the more water is removed. There are three different strengths: a 'strong' bag (3.86% glucose solution), a 'medium' bag (2.27% glucose) and a 'weak' bag (1.36% glucose). When there is too much water in the body (a condition called fluid overload, see *page 18*) the patient will be advised to use more strong or medium bags. These will remove more water than weak bags.

The strength of the bag is different from the size of the bag. A strong bag has more glucose in it than a weak bag, but it is no larger. Patients are advised to consider the weak bag as their 'standard' bag, and to try to use a minimum number of strong bags.

Alternative dialysis fluids

There are a number of new 'special' dialysis fluids which are sometimes prescribed for patients with particular problems.

• **Icodextrin.** This fluid contains a glucose polymer (in which the glucose molecules are stuck together), rather than ordinary glucose. Icodextrin may be recommended for PD patients who are diabetic or overweight. This is because the glucose polymer in Icodextrin is less likely than ordinary glucose to be absorbed into the body to cause problems with sugar balance or weight gain.

Icodextrin has also been shown to benefit patients who have been on PD for a long time and whose peritoneums do not work very well for dialysis.

- **Amino acids.** Some other dialysis fluids use amino acids rather than glucose. As amino acids are the building blocks of protein, and as some of the amino acids are absorbed into the blood, it is thought that these dialysis fluids might also act as food supplements. It is claimed that dialysis fluids containing amino acids are useful for patients who do not eat well or who have malnutrition (see *Chapter 12* for information on diet).

- **Bicarbonate.** A bicarbonate-based dialysis fluid has been developed to help patients who have problems regulating the level of acid in their bodies.

LIVING WITH PD

Once people develop ESRF, they will have it for the rest of their lives. Without treatment – by PD, haemodialysis or a kidney transplant – people with ESRF will die within a few weeks. With treatment, they will be able to do all or most of the things they did before they became ill. PD does affect a person's lifestyle – especially because of the need for daily dialysis – but the limitations are often less of a problem than many people might expect.

- **Flexibility.** PD is a flexible treatment which can be performed almost anywhere. The dialysis supplies can be delivered to most parts of the world, and some APD machines are portable.

- **Responsibility and independence.** People on PD usually do their own dialysis, usually in their own homes. This gives many PD patients a greater sense of responsibility and independence than is possible for the majority of haemodialysis patients (who receive their dialysis from nurses or dialysis technicians in a hospital).

- **Sport and exercise.** Most types of sport and exercise are possible for people on PD. Even contact sports are possible (though not always recommended). PD patients who want to play sports such as rugby, judo and karate are advised to wear a protective belt around their abdomen.

- **Swimming/baths/showers.** Before a swim (or bath or shower), PD patients need to cover their PD catheter with a special plastic dressing, which they can get either from the hospital or their family doctor. After a swim (or bath or shower), patients should clean the exit site of their catheter and, whenever possible, should also do a fluid exchange.

- **Sexual activity.** Sex is very possible for people on PD. Some people may find it uncomfortable to have sex with the dialysis fluid in, but they can drain it out first and use a new bag afterwards. Patients on APD can have sex either off or on the machine (the connecting lead is very long).

DELIVERY AND STORAGE OF SUPPLIES

PD is performed by patients themselves in their own homes. They therefore need to have supplies of fluid delivered to them and to be able to store these supplies in a convenient place. The bags of dialysis fluid come in boxes of four or five, and so a month's supplies can be as many as forty boxes. These can be stored in a cupboard under the stairs, a spare bedroom, the shed or even the garage.

Most people receive a delivery of supplies once a month, though patients with very small houses or flats may be able to arrange fortnightly deliveries. The people who deliver the supplies deliver to many other dialysis patients and are specially recruited and trained to go into patients' homes. They will move the supplies to exactly where a patient wants them, and will even move boxes around so that fluid from previous deliveries gets used before the new stock.

POSSIBLE PROBLEMS WITH PD

PD is not always entirely trouble free. Patients may experience various psychological and physical problems:

• **Feelings of restriction.** Some kidney patients feel that PD is more restrictive than haemodialysis because it never goes away. PD patients have to do dialysis every day. Haemodialysis patients, on the other hand, do at least have some 'let up' from it – they do have 'days off'.

• **Body image problems.** Some PD patients do not like the way PD affects their appearance. The abdomen tends to get stretched by PD, giving it a rounded appearance. Young people in particular may be very conscious of their body shape, especially if they are slim. Keeping fit and doing exercises to strengthen the abdominal muscles will help.

The PD catheter can also cause body image problems. PD patients have to come to terms with the fact that they now have a plastic tube permanently protruding from their abdomen. Some people find this very difficult to cope with, feeling that they have been severely mutilated. They may also worry that the catheter might put off a sexual partner. (See *Chapter 13* for more information on the psychological aspects of kidney failure.)

• **Sexual problems.** Sexual problems – such as reduced sex drive, impotence, and problems with fertility – are common among people with kidney failure. However, not all kidney patients have sexual problems, and for those who do, a range of treatments is available (see *Chapter 14*).

• **Fluid overload.** The amount of 'used' fluid that is drained out of the body after PD is about 1.5 litres per day more than the amount of fresh dialysis fluid that is put in. This extra fluid – in effect, the PD patient's urine – does not increase in quantity however much the patient drinks. This means that PD patients have to restrict their drinking to avoid problems due to fluid overload (see *Chapter 3* for details).

• **Discomfort.** Some PD patients find that the dialysis fluid in their abdomen is uncomfortable. It may also lead to backache.

• **Wearing out.** The peritoneum does not actually 'wear out', but in a very small number of patients it may cease to be effective as a dialysis membrane.

POOR DRAINAGE

One of the most common problems with PD – especially among new PD patients – is poor drainage of the dialysis fluid. The PD catheter may become blocked with a substance called fibrin, which is a form of protein. It looks like tiny strands of cotton wool and is completely harmless. A patient may be able to clear the catheter simply by squeezing the tubing to dislodge the fibrin. Alternatively, a nurse will be able to clear the catheter by injecting water, saline (a salt solution) or a de-clotting agent, called heparin, down the catheter. This is a simple procedure and will not need an operation.

The most common reason for poor drainage is constipation. If a PD patient becomes constipated, the bowels press against the catheter and make the dialysis fluid drain very slowly. The fluid may also get trapped in pockets of bowel, preventing it from draining properly. So, it is very important to avoid constipation, perhaps by taking regular laxatives.

Another reason for poor drainage is that the catheter is in the wrong position. Sometimes a displaced catheter will 'float' back into the right position naturally. If this does not happen, then an operation may be required to correct the position of the catheter.

Leaks

In most PD patients, the 'seal' around the catheter exit site (where the catheter leaves the abdomen) works properly. PD fluid drains in and out of the abdomen through the tube without any leakage. However, in some patients, the PD fluid leaks out around the catheter, wetting the dressing over the exit site.

If a leaking catheter is 'rested' (not used for dialysis) for 2 to 4 weeks, it will usually 'seal up' again, and become water-tight. Occasionally, however, a leak may recur even if the catheter is rested. It may then be necessary to have an operation to take out the leaking catheter. A new catheter, at a different site, is usually put in during the same operation.

In some men on PD, fluid leaks into the scrotum and causes swelling of the genitals. This is called a scrotal leak. If a scrotal leak occurs, PD must be stopped temporarily until the leak has healed.

Hernias

A hernia occurs when a wall of muscle weakens and lets an organ or tissue out from inside. Hernias can cause difficulties for PD patients. If a patient has a hernia before the PD catheter is put in, it can become more of a problem afterwards. The daily draining of PD fluid into and out of the abdomen can cause the hernia to become bigger (and more painful).

If nothing is done, the bowel can become 'stuck' inside the hernia, thereby blocking the bowel. This will require an emergency operation. If an existing hernia is noticed by the surgeon during an operation to insert a PD catheter, it will be repaired during the same operation to stop it causing problems in the future.

Peritonitis

Peritonitis is an infection of the peritoneum. It is usually caused by one of two types of bacteria (called *staphylococcus epidermidis* and *staphylococcus aureus).* In rare but serious cases, peritonitis in PD patients is caused by a fungus (usually a type called *candida albicans).*

The most common reason why PD patients get peritonitis is that they touch the connection between the bag of fluid and the catheter. However, even if PD exchanges are scrupulously clean, infection can still enter the abdomen from the outside world through the catheter. PD patients can expect to get on average less than one attack of peritonitis every year. So it is not that common. Indeed, some patients never get it. Patients on APD are less likely to get peritonitis than those on CAPD, probably because fewer catheter connections are required.

A patient will know when they have peritonitis because the dialysis fluid that drains out will be cloudy. This fluid is normally 'see-through'. Sometimes patients have abdominal pain and a fever as well – but not always. The treatment is simple and effective – usually one or more antibiotics to be added to the fresh dialysis fluid. Patients are shown how to do this – i.e., they treat peritonitis themselves in their own homes.

A patient will not be offered a transplant if a kidney becomes available during an attack of peritonitis.This is because the drugs that are given after a transplant to prevent kidney rejection (see *Chapter 10*) may make the peritonitis worse. These drugs, which are called immuno-suppressant drugs, make it harder for the body's immune (defence) system to fight any type of invader (including germs as well as transplanted organs).

Occasionally, a patient may get several attacks of peritonitis in a row. The doctor may then decide that an operation to replace the PD catheter is needed straight away. Alternatively, the doctor may decide that it is better to delay replacing the catheter and to 'rest' the abdomen by not using it for PD for a period of 4 to 6 weeks. If this happens, the patient will usually need to have haemodialysis until PD is resumed.

If peritonitis is caused by a fungus, it will be treated straight away – by an operation to remove the PD catheter. Drugs are not very effective against fungi, but the problem soon goes away if the catheter is removed. The catheter can still be replaced at a later date.

If a patient has many bad attacks of peritonitis, PD may no longer be suitable for them. They will then have to change to haemodialysis as their long-term treatment.

EXIT SITE INFECTIONS

PD patients may also get another type of infection, called an exit site infection. This causes a red tender area around the exit site (the point where the PD catheter comes out through the skin). Also, when someone has this type of infection, squeezing around the exit site may produce some pus.

Some PD patients get exit site infections regularly, whereas others never get them. Keeping the catheter taped down to the skin will help reduce the risk of an exit site infection, especially when the catheter is new.

Exit site infections respond well to antibiotics, usually given either as tablets or creams. Sometimes, a single intravenous injection of an antibiotic called *vancomycin* is needed. There is usually no need to remove the PD catheter.

Occasionally, an exit site infection spreads down the catheter 'tunnel' (the route taken by the catheter through the abdominal wall). This type of infection is called a tunnel infection. Antibiotics are not always effective when someone has a tunnel infection. An operation to remove the catheter will then be necessary. It is usually possible to insert a new catheter at the same operation.

KEY FACTS

1. In PD, the process of dialysis takes place inside the patient's abdomen.
2. PD is suitable for most people with ESRF.
3. The patient's peritoneum (abdominal lining) acts as the dialysis membrane.
4. Dialysis fluid from a bag is drained into the peritoneal cavity, left there until dialysis has taken place, and is then drained out.
5. Patients are trained to do PD themselves, in their own homes.
6. One advantage of PD is the independence it gives to patients.
7. Storage space in the home is needed to accommodate bulky supplies of dialysis fluid.
8. Peritonitis is the main problem with PD. Patients know they have peritonitis when their used dialysis fluid becomes cloudy.

9 HAEMODIALYSIS

This chapter describes haemodialysis, which is the traditional type of dialysis used to treat people with chronic kidney failure.

INTRODUCTION

Haemodialysis is the older of the two types of dialysis. This treatment became available in the 1960s, and since then has enabled large numbers of kidney patients to lead almost normal lives. The main difference between haemodialysis and the other type of dialysis – called peritoneal dialysis or PD (see *Chapter 8*) – is that in haemodialysis, the process of dialysis (see *Chapter 7*) takes place outside the body, in a machine.

WHO CAN BE TREATED BY HAEMODIALYSIS?

Almost all patients with end-stage renal failure (ESRF) can be treated by haemodialysis. The only real requirements are:

- It must be possible to gain good access to a patient's bloodstream (see *page 50*). (Access can be a particular problem for kidney patients who have diabetes, *see page 56*.)
- Patients must be able to withstand major changes in blood pressure and toxin levels. (Most people have no problems with this, but some patients with heart problems are unable to cope.)

WHAT DOES HAEMODIALYSIS DO?

Haemodialysis takes over some of the work that the kidneys can no longer manage when someone has kidney failure. Like PD, haemodialysis removes the waste products of food (toxin clearance, see *Chapter 2*) and it removes excess water from the body (see *Chapter 3*). It can also be used to give people with kidney failure various substances that they may be short of, such as bicarbonate and calcium.

Either haemodialysis or PD can provide dialysis that is equivalent to about 5% of the work done by two healthy kidneys. This is enough to relieve most of the symptoms of kidney failure and to enable people to do all, or most of, the things they could do before they became ill.

HOW DOES HAEMODIALYSIS WORK?

The basic principles of dialysis – which apply to both haemodialysis and PD – are explained in detail in *Chapter 7*. Briefly, both types of dialysis use a special liquid (called the dialysis fluid, dialysis solution or dialysate) and a membrane (called the dialysis membrane) to do some of the work of the kidneys.

In haemodialysis, the process of dialysis occurs in a machine. This machine is called a dialysis machine or kidney machine (see *top diagram*). Blood from the patient is pumped through the machine so that dialysis can take place. Dialysis fluid and water are also pumped through the machine.

The dialysis machine contains a special filtering unit called the dialyser or artificial kidney (see *bottom diagram*). The dialyser is a cylinder that contains thousands of very small hollow tubes. Each of the tubes is made from very thin plastic, which acts as the dialysis membrane. The patient's blood is pumped through the middle of the tubes. Meanwhile, the dialysis fluid is pumped around the outside of the tubes. The process of dialysis takes place through tiny holes in the tubes. Various substances and water can easily pass through the holes, but blood cells cannot.

During dialysis, body wastes (such as creatinine and urea) pass from the blood into the dialysis fluid. They do this by a process called diffusion, by which substances pass from a stronger to a weaker solution (see *pages 35-36*.) Meanwhile other substances that are needed by the body (such as bicarbonate and calcium) can be supplied to them from the dialysis fluid. Again, it is diffusion (now working in the opposite direction) that makes this possible.

The second main function of the kidneys (and therefore of dialysis) is to remove water. The way that this is done in haemodialysis is not the same as in PD. (In PD, water is removed by a process called osmosis, see *page 36*). In haemodialysis, it is the action of the dialysis machine that removes the water. The machine applies a sucking pressure that draws water out of the blood and into the dialysis fluid. This process is known as ultrafiltration (see also *page 36*) or 'u'...'f'...'ing'. Instructions about the amount of water to be removed and the rate of ultrafiltration are entered into the machine at the start of each dialysis session.

How a dialysis (kidney) machine works

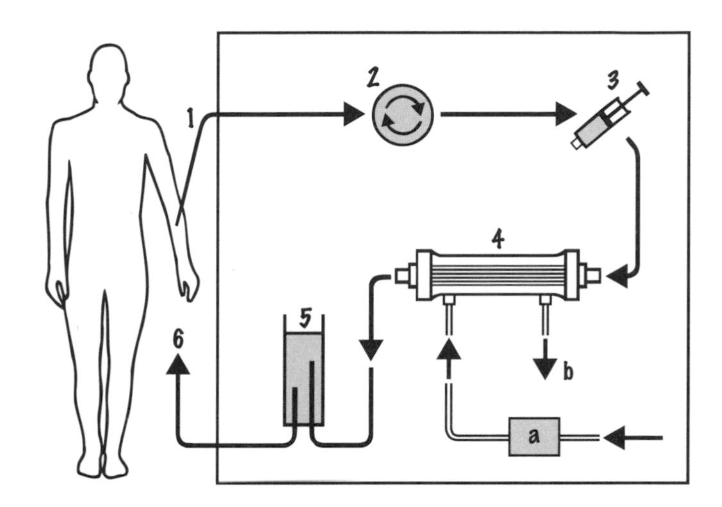

1 Blood comes from the arm
2 Blood is pumped to the machine
3 Heparin (a blood thinning drug) is added to the blood
4 Blood enters the dialyser. Dialysis fluid with treated water (a) enters the dialyser, and wastes are taken away to a drain (b)
5 Blood passes through a bubble trap
6 Blood goes back to the arm

A dialyser (artificial kidney)

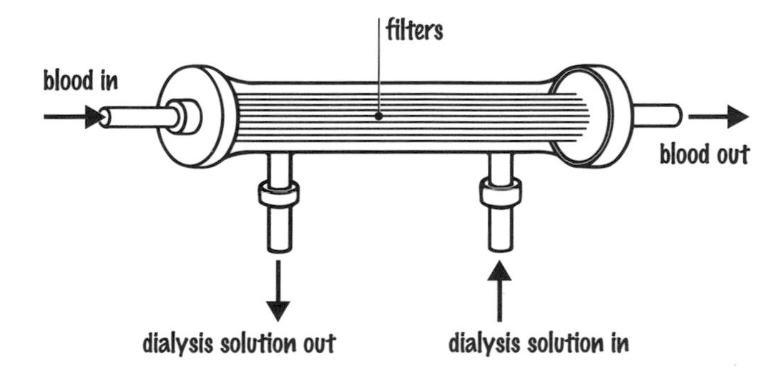

DIFFERENT DIALYSERS AND MACHINES

There are many sorts of dialysers available and different renal units tend to have their own preferences. Although the dialysers may look quite different from one another, the way in which they work is the same. The same applies to dialysis machines. Manufacturers opt for different colour schemes and shapes. Also, different machines display information in different ways, but they all tell much the same story.

HOW IS HAEMODIALYSIS DONE?

To do haemodialysis, the patient must be connected to a dialysis machine. The machine may be in a hospital renal unit, in a satellite dialysis unit or, less commonly, in the patient's own home (see *pages 53-54*).

Haemodialysis is done by taking blood from the body and pumping it around a dialysis machine and through a dialyser. In the dialyser, toxins and excess water – which are the equivalent of the urine produced by healthy kidneys – pass from the blood into the dialysis fluid. The cleansed blood is then returned to the body at the same rate at which it is removed. Meanwhile, the 'used' dialysis fluid (full of toxins and extra water) is pumped out of the dialysis machine and down the drain.

Haemodialysis is usually done three times a week, for 3 to 5 hours each session. The exact length of the sessions will depend on the amount of waste that an individual patient produces; bigger people generally need longer dialysis sessions than smaller people. Longer sessions may also be needed by patients who do not pass any urine.

Most renal units use a new dialyser at each dialysis session, but some units – especially in the United States – clean the dialysers after use and re-use them several times on the same patient.

'ACCESS' TO THE BLOODSTREAM

The term 'access' soon becomes familiar to patients on haemodialysis. It refers to the method by which access is gained to the bloodstream so that dialysis can take place.

During haemodialysis, large quantities of blood must be rapidly removed from the body and just as rapidly returned to it (at the same time). Therefore, in most cases, access has two 'sides'. One of these (often called the 'arterial side') is used to take blood out of the patient's body. The other (often called the 'venous side') is used to return blood to the patient after dialysis.

There are two main types of access:

- a dialysis catheter, which is usually a double-barrelled plastic tube (see *below*); and
- a fistula, which is formed from the patient's own blood vessels by joining a vein to an artery (see *page 52*).

DIALYSIS CATHETERS

A haemodialysis catheter is a plastic tube, usually with two separate barrels, one for removing blood from the body, and the other for returning it after dialysis. The catheter, which needs to be half in and half out of the body, is inserted during a short operation. This operation may be performed under either a general or a local anaesthetic. The catheter is inserted into a large vein either at the side of the neck, under the collarbone, or at the top of the leg next to the groin (see *diagram, next page*). Names sometimes used for catheters in these different places are a 'jugular line' (at the side of the neck), a 'subclavian line' (under the collarbone), and a 'femoral line' (in the groin).

Dialysis catheters may be temporary or permanent. Temporary catheters are often used while patients are waiting for a fistula to be created. Other patients – particularly those with diabetes – have blood vessels that are not strong enough for a fistula, and will need a permanent catheter for haemodialysis access.

Permanent catheters are tunnelled deeper under the skin than temporary catheters. They also have small cuffs around them, just under the skin, to help keep them in place, and to help keep germs out of the body.

Entry positions for haemodialysis catheter lines

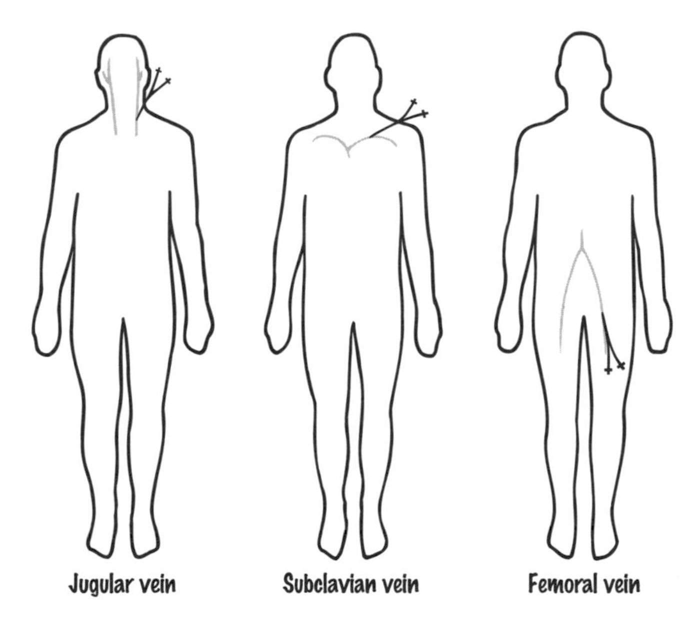

Permanent catheters also tend to be softer and more flexible than most temporary catheters.

After each dialysis session, saline (salt dissolved in water) is injected into the line to remove any blood. The inside of the catheter is then filled with a drug called heparin. Heparin stops the formation of blood clots, which could block the catheter. This keeps the catheter clear of clots between dialysis sessions. Access is the haemodialysis patient's lifeline, and catheters must always be treated with great care by doctors, nurses and patients. Between dialysis sessions, patients are asked to keep their catheter clean and dry, and to ensure that it has a dressing on it at all times.

FISTULAS

The usual form of access for haemodialysis is the arteriovenous fistula or AVF (often simply called a fistula). Fistulas are made by a surgeon in a small operation, which may be performed under a general or a local anaesthetic. In this operation (see *diagram, next page*), a vein (a blood vessel that carries blood back to the heart) is joined to an artery (a blood vessel that carries blood away from the heart). This can be done under the skin, usually at either the wrist or the elbow.

The blood pressure in arteries is always higher than the blood pressure in veins. When a fistula is formed, blood from the artery flows into the vein, and causes it to enlarge a little. Once the fistula has 'matured' (i.e., grown), it will be ready for dialysis. This usually takes about six weeks.

Whenever a fistula is used for haemodialysis, a local anaesthetic may be applied to the area and then two large needles are inserted into the fistula. These needles provide access to the bloodstream for dialysis, and are removed at the end of the session. Fistulas are a better form of access than catheters because they do not use any plastic, and so are less likely to become infected.

The creation of a fistula means that some blood that would normally have gone to the hand (or arm) in the artery used for the fistula, instead bypasses the hand or arm and goes up the fistula. This does not normally cause any problems. However, occasionally, the hand or arm becomes cold and painful because of the blood that is 'stolen' from it by the fistula. This is called steal syndrome. Severe steal syndrome may mean that the fistula has to be 'tied off' – i.e., permanently blocked off by a surgeon during another small operation.

When a fistula is touched, a buzzing sensation is felt. This is known as a bruit (pronounced 'broo-ee'). Patients with fistulas are advised to check for the buzz every day. They should do this gently as fistulas can be fragile.

If there is no buzz when a fistula is touched, this probably means that the fistula has become blocked by a blood clot. Often this occurs at night and is caused by accidentally sleeping on the fistula arm. If no buzz can be felt, it is important to contact the hospital as soon as possible – as it may be possible to clear the clot and save the fistula.

A fistula

1 Normal vein

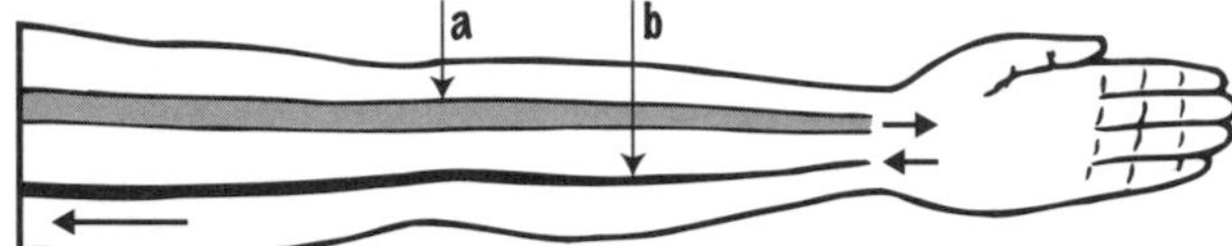

a Artery takes blood to the arm and hand
b Vein takes blood from the hand and arm

2 Vein diversion

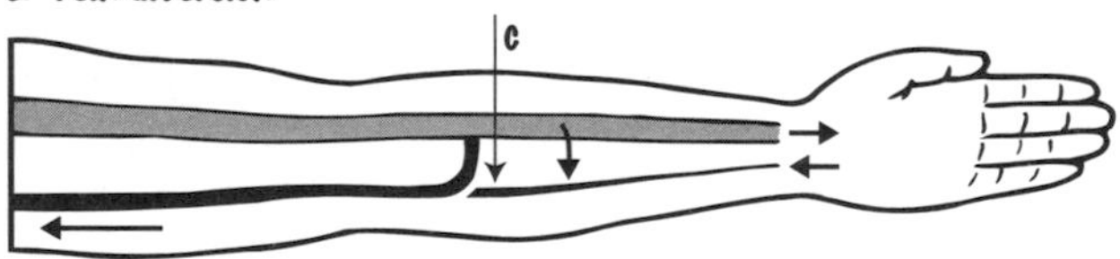

c A diversion of the vein is formed, linking it to the artery in the forearm

3 Vein thickens

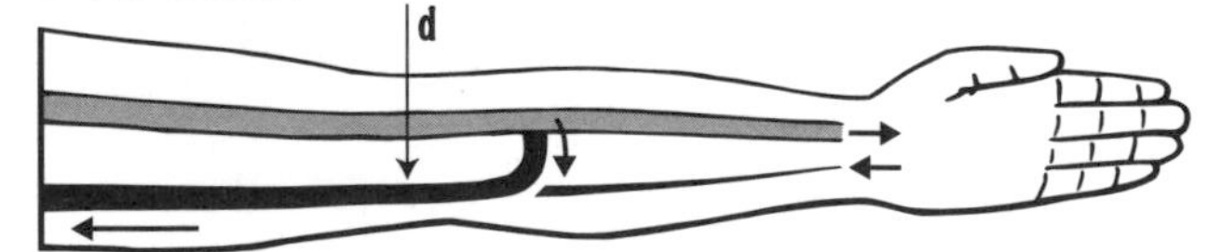

d The vein thickens beyond the link, and can now be used as a fistula

OTHER TYPES OF ACCESS

There are other types of access available, which are used when the two main types (double-barrelled catheters and fistulas) no longer work. This usually happens in patients with fragile blood vessels.

- **Grafts.** A graft is a plastic connecting tube that joins an artery to a vein, inside the patient's arm or leg. (It is therefore different from a fistula, in which the patient's artery and vein are joined directly without a plastic connector.) The graft must be inserted by a surgeon during an operation. Grafts are made of a special self-sealing material (for example, Gortex) through which dialysis needles can be inserted. A graft can be used many hundreds of times.

- **Single-barrelled catheters.** It is sometimes necessary to use a single-barrelled catheter. This is inserted into the same sites that would have been used for a double-barrelled catheter.

SINGLE-NEEDLE DIALYSIS

It is also possible to do haemodialysis using a single needle to remove and return the blood (rather than the two needles used for 'normal' dialysis). The single needle is inserted into a fistula or a graft. Alternatively, a single-barrelled catheter can be used. Single-needle dialysis is sometimes used for patients who have developing fistulas or grafts, or if a patient's fistula never enlarges properly.

HOW MUCH DIALYSIS IS NEEDED?

In most hospitals it is the nurses in the renal unit who are responsible for working out how long kidney patients need to spend on the dialysis machine, and also what size of dialyser they will use. There are different sizes of dialyser – bigger ones remove more toxins than smaller ones. Longer dialysis sessions will also remove more toxins.

As a rule, the bigger/more muscular the patient, the more dialysis they will need. In order to change the amount of dialysis that a patient receives, the nurse can choose to alter the size of the dialyser and/or the length of time that the patient spends on the machine.

The dialysis dose can be worked out simply by comparing the levels of wastes (such as urea or creatinine) in the patient's blood before and after dialysis (see *Chapter 2* for details), and making sure that there is a significant reduction. Some units still use this method, but it is now more common to use one of the newer methods of working out dialysis doses. The first of these uses a calculation called the urea reduction ratio, the other is a method called urea kinetic modelling (UKM). With each of these methods, dialysis target figures are the same whatever the size of the patient.

The urea reduction ratio is really just a more formal way of comparing urea levels in the blood before and after dialysis. As before, the patient's urea levels are measured in millimoles per litre (mmol/l) of blood, but now the measurements before and after dialysis are used to calculate a percentage reduction in blood urea. (For example, if the blood urea before dialysis was 30 mmol/l, and after dialysis it was 15 mmol/l, then the percentage reduction in urea during dialysis was 50%.) Such information allows adjustments to be made at future dialysis sessions in order to achieve the current urea reduction target of at least 65% per session.

Urea kinetic modelling also compares the levels of urea in the patient's blood before and after dialysis. However, this method also takes into account the size of the dialyser (called 'K'), the time the patient will need on the machine (called 't') and a number that reflects the patient's body weight (called 'V'). This produces a figure called the Kt/V (pronounced 'K...t...over V'). Because a patient's Kt/V figure refers to the amount of urea cleared from the body, the higher the number the better (see also *page 14*). Recent recommendations state that Kt/V should be more than 1.2 for each dialysis session.

Some patients on haemodialysis believe that it is the amount of fluid that needs to be removed which determines the length of time that they must spend on the dialysis machine. This is wrong. The most important factor affecting the length of dialysis is the amount of toxins that needs to be removed. However, if a patient has a lot of fluid to remove, they may need to spend extra time on the machine to achieve this.

HAEMODIALYSIS IN HOSPITAL

Most haemodialysis patients receive their treatment in a specially designed renal (kidney) unit within a hospital. This is called unit haemodialysis.

Patients attend the hospital, usually three times a week, to use one of the unit's dialysis machines. Unlike PD (see *Chapter 8*), in which patients have almost total responsibility for their dialysis, unit haemodialysis still tends to be done on behalf of the patient, by nurses, healthcare assistants and technicians. Patients therefore have very little responsibility for their dialysis sessions – other than turning up at the right time. This may suit some patients for various personal and medical reasons.

For other patients, however, the lack of control over their own treatment is not satisfactory. To address this problem, many hospital renal units now encourage their more able patients to become involved in their own care. This may mean simply having patients check their own blood pressure before dialysis, but it may go as far as teaching patients to put themselves on to, and taking themselves off, the dialysis machine.

Visiting the hospital three times a week for haemodialysis sessions does have its advantages. It helps patients to avoid the feelings of isolation that may occur when dialysis is done at home (either PD or home haemodialysis, see *below*). Unit dialysis also gives patients with ESRF frequent and regular access to medical and nursing expertise, education and support, as well as an opportunity to chat to other patients who are 'in the same boat'.

SATELLITE HAEMODIALYSIS

A few hospitals now offer what is called satellite haemodialysis. This takes place away from the main hospital, in a 'satellite unit'. At the satellite unit, a small number of the hospital's healthier patients are treated by relatively few nurses. The patients generally do some of the dialysis preparation themselves. This allows patients to feel more in control of their treatment than is often possible in hospital-based units.

Satellite units can be more convenient for patients as they tend to be nearer to residential areas than many hospital buildings, making them more accessible by car or public transport. It may also be possible to arrange haemodialysis sessions after normal working hours.

HAEMODIALYSIS AT HOME

Some kidney patients can do haemodialysis in their own homes. The dialysis machines used today have many safety devices built into them, so it is usually quite safe to dialyse at home. This is called home haemodialysis.

Whether or not a patient can have home haemodialysis depends partly on the hospital and partly on the patient. Some renal units are more willing than others to provide home haemodialysis. Even if a unit is willing, the money must be available to supply the dialysis machine, to convert a room in the patient's home to be used for dialysis and to put in a special water supply.

To be considered for home dialysis, patients must:

- be quite fit, with no access problems;
- be able to learn to do dialysis, and be able to solve the various problems that might occur during a dialysis session;
- have someone around to help every time they are on the machine.

As long as these conditions are met, home haemodialysis can be an ideal option for kidney patients who value their independence and who perhaps need to fit in haemodialysis around a busy work schedule.

LIVING WITH HAEMODIALYSIS

The need to do haemodialysis three times a week does have an effect on lifestyle. Having to make frequent trips to the hospital can be an irritation and may interfere with the patient's family or work life. Home haemodialysis may be less disruptive, but still involves a long-term regular commitment to the treatment by the patient and other members of the family.

Doing haemodialysis can restrict a kidney patient's holiday choices. Holidays can sometimes be difficult to arrange because of the need for patients to find a dialysis centre that is willing to treat them while they are away from home.

Haemodialysis patients are less likely than PD patients to have body image worries. Some haemodialysis patients need a permanent catheter to provide access, and they may feel unhappy about the effect this has on their appearance. However, the more usual form of access for haemodialysis is the fistula, which is much less visible. (See *Chapter 13* for more information about the psychological aspects of kidney failure.)

Possible problems during haemodialysis

Haemodialysis, like all medical procedures, is not without its problems. Most of the problems that occur with haemodialysis are related to the speed with which water is removed from the bloodstream during dialysis. Removing water from the bloodstream quickly is a bit like letting air out of a balloon. When air is released from a balloon, the pressure inside it drops, and it becomes less rigid. In humans, when water is let out of the blood over a short period of time, the blood pressure falls.

Haemodialysis is a more 'aggressive' form of dialysis than PD. In haemodialysis, all the dialysis is crammed into three sessions a week, each one lasting only 3 to 5 hours. In other words, the balloon is let down very quickly. The rapid changes in blood pressure (usually a fall), and in the blood levels of water and body wastes that occur during a haemodialysis session, can make some patients feel quite unwell, either during or after the session. Fainting, vomiting, cramps, temporary loss of vision, chest pain, fatigue and irritability can all occur.

The best way to avoid problems caused by rapid physical changes during haemodialysis is for patients to stick to recommended fluid intake limits. For most haemodialysis patients, the recommended daily fluid intake is about 1 litre of fluid. (PD patients can usually have 1.5 litres.)

Some renal units use a technique called sodium profiling to prevent problems caused by the rapid removal of water. However, not all kidney doctors and nurses agree that this is useful. Although sodium profiling does help in the removal of fluid and does stop dizziness and cramps during dialysis, it may also make patients more thirsty after dialysis – and so more likely to need more fluid removing at the next dialysis session. For this reason, some people believe that sodium profiling creates a vicious circle of excessive drinking and fluid removal.

Fluid overload and haemodialysis

Between dialysis sessions, haemodialysis patients sometimes develop the condition called fluid overload (see *page 17* for details). This causes excess fluid to collect first in the skin at the ankles and then elsewhere in the body, including the lungs.

Problems with fluid overload are usually due to drinking too much. However, the problem is not always the patient's fault. It can also occur when the person in charge of a dialysis session does not set the controls to take off enough fluid, or misjudges a patient's dry weight.

If a patient between dialysis sessions thinks that they may have fluid overload, they should contact the hospital at once. It may be necessary for them to have an extra dialysis session to remove the excess fluid. Constantly being fluid overloaded causes the blood pressure to rise. Like a balloon which contains too much air, the heart muscle stretches, and will eventually weaken.

The best way for patients to avoid the complications associated with fluid overload is to stick to the fluid restrictions they have been given.

Hyperkalaemia (excess potassium)

Another problem that may occur between haemodialysis sessions is called hyperkalaemia. This means that there is too much potassium in the blood (also *see Chapter 12*).

A raised level of potassium in the blood may cause the heart to flutter, and even stop. Hyperkalaemia can be very dangerous. It requires urgent medical treatment, and sometimes immediate dialysis. If hyperkalaemia is a problem for a patient on haemodialysis, they will be asked to restrict their intake of foods that contain a lot of potassium.

PROBLEMS WITH ACCESS

There may also be problems with the different types of haemodialysis access.

The usual type of haemodialysis access is a fistula (see *above, page 51*). If a fistula works well, it makes haemodialysis technically easy. However, not all fistulas work perfectly. Some never develop into a vein that is large enough for the blood flow to be adequate. Some function for months or even years, then suddenly stop working. In either case, a surgeon will then have to make a new fistula (or sometimes a graft) in another part of the body. Unfortunately, there are only a certain number of veins that are suitable to be used in this way. If patients require haemodialysis for many years, they may eventually run out of suitable veins.

To use a fistula (or graft), it is necessary to insert needles into it at the start of each dialysis session. Even with a local anaesthetic, some patients find this painful.

Because of the limited 'life' of fistulas, grafts and dialysis catheters, haemodialysis may eventually become impossible. This can be a particular problem for patients with diabetes mellitus (sugar diabetes).

Dialysis catheters may also cause problems. Some patients find it difficult to cope with their changed body image (see also *Chapter 13*). Another problem is that dialysis catheters sometimes stop working because they have become blocked by a blood clot. If a catheter stops working, it will have to be replaced. Again, as for fistulas and grafts, there are only a certain number of veins suitable for plastic tubes. Dialysis catheters are more likely to become infected than either fistulas or grafts.

PROBLEMS FOR DIABETICS

The blood vessels of people with diabetes are often very narrow. This can make it almost impossible to form a fistula in some patients. Inserting plastic tubes into the veins can also be very difficult. For this reason, many doctors recommend PD rather than haemodialysis for kidney patients with diabetes.

There is also a fear that the drug heparin, which is normally given during haemodialysis to prevent blood clotting, can cause bleeding at the back of the eye. By the time they need dialysis, most diabetics with kidney failure are prone to this type of bleeding (a condition called diabetic retinopathy), which can cause blindness. It may therefore be better to avoid having to use heparin.

However, not all doctors think that haemodialysis is not a good option for kidney patients with diabetes. Some consider that haemodialysis is just as good as PD for this group of patients, does not worsen vision and may even have some advantages.

BLEEDING

Haemodialysis patients may have problems with bleeding either during a dialysis session or, more commonly, after dialysis when the fistula needles are removed. Sometimes bleeding can result from using heparin during dialysis. So most centres now try to use as little heparin as possible, and some people have heparin-free dialysis. To try to stop the bleeding after dialysis, it is common for the heparin to be turned off at least one hour before the end of the dialysis session.

INFECTIONS

There is always a risk that a patient will pick up an infection during a dialysis session. Germs may enter the patient's blood either from the haemodialysis access or from the lines of the machine. During sessions of dialysis, fevers often become worse and there may be rigors (shivering attacks).

Infections can usually be treated with antibiotics, but it is better to avoid getting an infection in the first place. This can be achieved by strict attention to hygiene. Care is needed both with personal hygiene and when the dialysis machine and access lines are set up. Fistulas are much less likely to get infected than dialysis catheters.

Patients may sometimes develop an infection where the haemodialysis catheter comes out from under the skin. This is called an exit site infection, and causes the area around the catheter to become sore and inflamed. Most exit site infections respond well to antibiotics.

The inside of the catheter can also become infected. This is called a line infection, and can make patients very unwell, causing fever and rigors. If a patient develops a line infection, their catheter will usually be removed and replaced after the fever has settled. Temporary catheters are more likely to become infected than permanent ones, and for this reason temporary catheters should be replaced after about three weeks of use even if they are not obviously infected. This helps to prevent line infections.

KEY FACTS

1. In haemodialysis, the process of dialysis takes place inside a machine.
2. Haemodialysis is suitable for most people with kidney failure.
3. In a haemodialysis session, blood is taken from the body, pumped into the dialysis machine, cleaned by an artificial kidney (dialyser), and pumped back into the body .
4. Haemodialysis is usually done three times a week, each session lasting 3 to 5 hours.
5. In order to do haemodialysis, it is necessary to gain direct access to the patient's bloodstream. The usual types of access are a dialysis catheter or a fistula (made by joining a vein to an artery).
6. Most patients have haemodialysis in a hospital, but some have it in a satellite dialysis unit or at home.
7. Some patients may feel sick or dizzy during a haemodialysis session. This is usually due to the rapid removal of water and toxins, which results in a rapid drop in blood pressure.
8. Haemodialysis patients have a stricter fluid restriction than PD patients.
9. Because of the limited 'life' of fistulas, grafts and dialysis catheters, haemodialysis may eventually become impossible for some patients.

10 TRANSPLANTATION

This chapter provides information about the various procedures that are necessary before a patient can have a kidney transplant. It then describes what happens during the operation, and what to expect after the transplant has taken place.

INTRODUCTION

A successful kidney transplant is a more effective treatment for kidney failure than either peritoneal dialysis (see *Chapter 8*) or haemodialysis (see *Chapter 9*). However, not all patients are suitable for transplantation, and not all suitable patients are suitable all the time. Also, before a transplant can take place, it is necessary to find an appropriate donor kidney, which may not be easy. The first kidney transplant operations were performed in the 1950s. The operation itself is straightforward, with a good success rate. After a transplant, patients will need to take drugs daily for the rest of their lives. If a transplant fails, patients can go back to dialysis or possibly have another transplant.

THE BENEFITS

A kidney transplant can deliver the best quality of life to people with end-stage renal failure (ESRF). There is no doubt that for the right patient at the right time, a transplant is the best treatment option. A 'good' transplant provides about 50% of the function of two normal kidneys (compared with only about 5% from either type of dialysis).

The most obvious advantage of a transplant to people with kidney failure is freedom from dialysis. If a transplant works well, dialysis becomes a thing of the past. There are also no particular fluid or dietary restrictions after a transplant. Most people who have had a transplant feel better and have more energy than they did on dialysis. They are more able to cope with a job, and many find that their sex lives improve.

WHO CAN HAVE A TRANSPLANT?

Many patients with kidney failure are suitable for a transplant, provided a suitable donor kidney can be found (see *next page*). Patients who will probably not be considered suitable include anyone with serious heart disease or a serious type of cancer.

Most renal units do not have an age limit for kidney transplantation. Patients are considered on merit (i.e., their suitability for a transplant), rather than age. However, having said that, most units would think very seriously before transplanting a patient over 70 years old. Doctors do not believe that transplanting an older patient 'wastes' a kidney that a younger person would get 'more benefit' from. The main reason is that older patients often do not tolerate the transplant operation very well. Also, the drugs that are needed after a transplant (see *page 68*) are often too strong for older patients.

DO YOU HAVE TO BE ON DIALYSIS FIRST?

Most renal units will not put patients onto the national waiting list for a transplant kidney (see *page 62* for details) until they are stable on dialysis. However, a few units will put patients onto the list before this point. Also, if someone has a transplant that is failing, they may be put onto the list and given a new kidney before they have to go back on dialysis.

The national waiting list is for what is known as a cadaveric transplant (see *page 61*). This type of transplant uses a kidney that has been removed from someone who has died. Most of the transplant kidneys in the UK come from this source. The remainder are what are known as 'living related transplants' or LRTs (see *page 61*), or 'living unrelated transplants' (see *page 62*). For some patients, the possibility of obtaining a transplant kidney from a living donor will be the best chance of having a transplant operation before dialysis is needed.

Given that it is possible for people with kidney failure to be given a transplant before they need dialysis, you may wonder why don't all hospitals do it? The reason is that most doctors think that because there is such a shortage of kidneys for transplantation, it is better if patients all around the UK start waiting for a kidney at an equivalent time point, i.e., when they start dialysis. This makes it fair for everyone.

However, some renal units are undoubtedly better organised in terms of transplantation than others. So, some units do carry out transplants before dialysis. Some units also make more effort to obtain kidneys than others, and some units are keener on LRTs than others. For all these reasons, patients in some units may wait less time for a transplant, and are more likely to have a transplant before they need dialysis, than is usual in other units.

FINDING A SUITABLE KIDNEY

For a kidney transplant to be successful, it is essential that the tissues of the new kidney are fairly similar to the patient's original kidney. If the new kidney is not a good enough match, the patient's immune system (natural defence system) will attack and reject it. (See *page 66* for a description of the rejection process.)

Before a suitable kidney can be looked for, it is necessary for patients to have a number of tests. The most important of these are to find out the patient's blood group (see *below*) and tissue type (see *page 60*). The results will then be checked against the results of similar tests carried out either on an available kidney, or on a relative or other person who is considering donating one of their kidneys to the patient.

MATCHING THE BLOOD GROUP

The blood group is an inherited characteristic of red blood cells. It stays the same throughout your life. There are four main blood groups. These groups are called A, B, AB and O. Group O is the most common, followed by group A.

The blood group that you belong to depends on whether or not you have certain substances called antigens (types of protein) in your body. Two different antigens – called A and B – determine a person's blood group. If you have these antigens, they will be on the outer surface of all your cells, not just on your blood cells. If you have only antigen A, your blood group is A. If you have only antigen B, your blood group is B. If you have both antigen A and antigen B, your blood group is AB. If you have neither of these antigens, your blood group is O.

The function of the blood group antigens is to act as a 'friendly face' for the cells – so that the rest of the body can recognise the cells as their own, and leave them alone. A person's immune system will attack any cells that have a foreign antigen. This means that a patient can only be given a transplant kidney if the patient's and donor's blood groups are matched as follows:

Patient	Donor
Group O	Group O
Group A	Group A or group O
Group B	Group B or group O
Group AB	Any group (O, A, B, or AB)

MATCHING THE TISSUE TYPE

The principle of matching for tissue type is similar to that for matching for blood group. Again, the patient and the donor kidney or potential donor are matched using a blood test. The tissue typing test shows a person's genetic make-up (sometimes called their 'genetic fingerprint').

The tissue type is an inherited set of characteristics (antigens) on the surface of most cells. It stays the same throughout your life. You have only one tissue type (just as you only have one blood group), but your tissue type is made up of six different tissue type characteristics.

There are three main sorts of tissue type characteristic, called A, B and DR. Everyone has two of each (one from each parent) – making six in all. Just to make it more complicated, there are not only A, B and DR characteristics. In fact there are 20 or more different versions of each A, B and DR characteristic. This means that there are hundreds of different possible tissue types. So, for example, a tissue type could be A3/A7, B5/B9, DR3/DR21.

As there are so many possible tissue types, matching tissue types is a little more complicated than matching blood groups. However, basically, the more of these that are the same for the patient and the donor kidney or potential donor, the better the chances are that the transplant kidney will work.

Given the large number of tissue type possibilities, it is very unusual to get an exact match (called a '6 out of 6 match' or 'full-house match') between a patient and donor. Most units will offer a transplant if the patient and donor have three or more of the six tissue type characteristics in common. So, for example, a transplant might be offered in the following situation:

Patient:	**A3**/A7	B5/**B9**	**DR3**/DR21
Donor:	**A3**/A11	B1/**B9**	**DR3**/DR8

As the A3, B9 and DR3 characteristics are the same in this example. It would be called a '3 out of 6 match'.

The more characteristics that match the better. So a '6 out of 6 match' is better than a '3 out of 6 match'. The better the match, the more likely it is that the body will accept the kidney 'as its own', and not try to reject it. Unfortunately, it cannot be guaranteed that even a '6 out of 6' match will not be rejected. This is because the blood group and tissue type are not the only cell surface characteristics that are important. However, these other important characteristics have not all been identified.

TESTING FOR VIRUSES

Before a patient can be put forward for a transplant, they will have to be tested for various viruses. These include HIV (the virus that causes AIDS), hepatitis B, hepatitis C and cytomegalovirus (known as CMV). It is important to test for these viruses because they may be dormant ('sleeping', causing no symptoms) in a patient's body. After the transplant, they may be 'woken up' and cause illness.

If a patient refuses to have any of these tests, such as the HIV test, they will not be able to have a transplant. If a patient has one of the viruses, it does not mean that they will not get a transplant, it just means that the doctors will have to be more careful.

Other tests for transplant suitability

Other tests are also necessary before a patient can have a transplant. These include an electrocardiogram (ECG, an electric recording of the heart beat), and sometimes an echocardiogram (ECHO, a sound-wave picture of the heart) and a chest X-ray. Some renal units also insist that kidney patients who are diabetic also have a cardiac catheter test (a special X-ray picture of the heart).

If all the various test results are satisfactory, the patient can then be put on the national waiting list (see *page 62*) for a cadaveric transplant, or considered for a possible transplant from a living donor.

Cadaveric transplants

The term cadaveric transplant is used to describe a transplant kidney that has been removed from someone who has died. More than 90% of transplant kidneys in the UK come from this source.

Most of these donors have been killed in car accidents or died from a brain haemorrhage, and have been on a life support machine in an intensive care unit. Their kidneys can only be removed after they have been diagnosed 'brain dead'. This means that the part of the brain called the brainstem, which controls breathing, has stopped working permanently and that they are capable of living only if they are kept on a life support machine.

Kidneys for donation are usually removed when the donor's heart is still beating. For this reason, these donors are sometimes called heart-beating donors. Even though the heart is still beating, they would not breathe if they were not on a life support machine. Their brain is dead, and they have no chance of recovery.

Because of the shortage of donors, some renal units are obtaining transplant kidneys from people whose hearts have stopped beating. These donors – called non-heart-beating donors – are people who have died very suddenly, usually from a heart attack. Their hearts have stopped beating and they are brain dead. They have not been put on a life-support machine.

Kidneys from non-heart-beating donors are generally not as good as those from heart-beating donors. If you are offered a transplant, you can ask whether it is from a heart-beating or non-heart-beating donor. You have the right to know this, though you will not be told any other details about the donor.

If someone is on the national waiting list (see *page 62*) for a cadaveric kidney, they can still ask a relative, partner or friend to give them a kidney.

Living related transplants

Even though a cadaveric transplant is by far the most common type of kidney transplant in the UK, it is possible for patients to receive a kidney from a living relative. A growing number of renal units now have a transplant co-ordinator whose main job is to organise living related transplants (LRTs).

A living related transplant is 'better' than a cadaveric transplant, in that it is more likely to work. The best donor is an identical twin, as the tissue type is identical. Unfortunately, most people do not have an identical twin waiting to give them a kidney! Fortunately, a kidney from another relative may be suitable.

If a kidney patient has a relative who is at least 18 years old, healthy, and willing to give them a kidney, they should speak to the transplant coordinator (or other senior nurse, or doctor) at their unit. The most suitable donor is usually a brother, sister, father, mother, son or daughter, but other more distant relatives are sometimes suitable. As human beings do not need two kidneys to be healthy, the donor is unlikely to come to any harm by losing a kidney. However, even if a kidney comes from a close relative, it is important that both the donor and the patient understand that the kidney is not guaranteed to work.

It is up to kidney patients to ask their relatives to see if they are willing to donate a kidney. Doctors will not usually ask a patient's relatives for them, but they will talk to anybody who is willing to donate a kidney.

To find out if a relative is a suitable donor, it will be necessary for them to have the same blood tests as the patient, i.e., blood group, tissue type and virus tests. If they 'pass' this hurdle, they will then need to have further tests to check that their own kidneys are working perfectly. These include an ultrasound (a sound-wave picture) of the kidneys or an intravenous pyelogram (a type of X-ray that uses a special dye, given by injection, to show the drainage system of the kidneys). The final test is usually an arteriogram (also called an angiogram) of the blood vessels of the kidneys. This is a special type of X-ray taken after a substance that shows up on X-rays has been injected into a *catheter* in the groin). Some units do a CT scan instead of an arteriogram.

LRTs can be arranged before a patient starts dialysis. The tests described above can be organised in less than three months. But both sides – patient/donor and renal unit – need to move quickly to do this. Both the patient and the donor must make a lot of time available to get all the tests done, even if it means taking time off work.

Living unrelated transplants

It is not essential for a person who donates a kidney to be related to the patient. Kidneys may also be donated by someone close to the patient, such as a husband, wife, partner or good friend. This is called a living unrelated transplant.

Before a living unrelated transplant can take place, agreement must be obtained from a government body called ULTRA (Unrelated Live Transplantation Regulatory Authority). This process can slightly delay the transplant arrangements, which may therefore mean that they take longer than those for an LRT.

Kidney patients and potential donors are both advised to think very carefully before going ahead with transplantation from any living person. They need to consider very carefully what the emotional consequences might be if the transplant is not successful.

Xenotransplantation

The term xenotransplantation refers to the possibility of using organs (such as kidneys) taken from animals (especially pigs) for transplantation into humans. A certain amount of research has been done in this area, but the problems are currently considered to be too great. One major concern is the risk of passing on animal viruses to humans.

The transplant waiting list

At present, not enough cadaveric kidneys are donated to meet the demand. Changes in seat-belt laws and improvements in medicine mean that fewer people now die from the accidents or illnesses that would have made them suitable donors.

People who are waiting for a cadaveric kidney are

therefore put on a waiting list. Their details, including their blood group and tissue type, are put onto a national computer at the United Kingdom Transplant Support Service Authority (UKTSSA) in Bristol. When surgeons remove two kidneys from a patient who has died, one kidney is kept for patients dialysed in the area in which the patient died. The other is offered to the UKTSSA, which finds the most suitable patient for that kidney in the rest of the country.

The waiting list works on the basis of finding the 'right' dialysis patient for the 'right' kidney, when one becomes available. It does not work on a 'first-come-first-served' basis. Transplants are allocated to the patient who is the best match for the kidney in terms of blood group and tissue type. In other words, the patient does not join a queue, knowing that his or her name will come up after a reasonably fixed time. The average waiting time for a transplant is about two years. It is important to note that this is an average – it can be two days, or ten years.

It may sometimes be necessary to take a patient off the transplant list, either temporarily or permanently. This may be done, for example, if someone develops a serious infection or a heart problem, or if they need a major operation. This decision is not made lightly. Any patient who is being removed from the list should be told about the decision, and informed whether removal from the list is temporary or permanent. If a patient is unsure whether they are 'on the list', they should ask.

BEING READY FOR A TRANSPLANT

Patients who are on the waiting list for a transplant may not be given very much notice that a kidney is available for them. So, they need to be prepared to go to the hospital at short notice. Some patients are given a 'bleep' so that they can be contacted more easily.

When patients are on the transplant waiting list, it is largely up to them to make themselves contactable at all times, day and night. If a patient cannot be found, the kidney will be offered to someone else. When a patient 'gets the call', they should go to the hospital at once and not have anything to eat or drink (in preparation for the anaesthetic).

TESTS BEFORE THE OPERATION

Patients called in to the hospital for a transplant are not guaranteed to receive it. Before the operation can go ahead, it is necessary to check that the patient is well enough to have the operation, and that they will not reject the transplant kidney.

1. Physical examination. The patient is first given a thorough physical examination by a doctor. The purpose of this is to check that it is safe to proceed with the operation. For example, if a patient has a heavy cold, it may considered too much of a risk for them to have an anaesthetic. If the patient 'fails' this assessment, they will be sent home, and put back on the waiting list.

2. The cross-match. This test is the final hurdle before the operation. The cross-match is a blood test that checks the patient has no antibodies (substances that normally help the body to fight infection) that would react with the donor kidney. High levels of such antibodies in the blood mean that the new kidney is likely to be rejected as soon as it is put into the patient, even if it seems a good match.

A cross-match is done by mixing a sample of the patient's blood with cells from the donor's lymph nodes or spleen. If there is no reaction (i.e., the patient's blood does not start attacking the donor's cells), it is assumed that the patient will be less likely to reject the new kidney when it is transplanted. This is called a negative cross-match, and means that the operation can go ahead.

If the cross-match is positive (i.e., there is a reaction between the patient's blood and the donor's cells), the patient will be sent home, and put back on the waiting list. This can be very disappointing, but it is much better to return to dialysis for a while than to be given a kidney that doesn't work and which may make the recipient extremely ill.

THE TRANSPLANT OPERATION

An operation to transplant a kidney requires a general anaesthetic and lasts about two to three hours. The surgeon makes a diagonal incision (cut) into the abdomen, on the right or the left, below the navel (see *diagram 1, facing page*).

The patient's own kidneys are usually left in place. The transplant kidney is placed lower down in the abdomen, just above the groin (see *diagram 2*). The transplant kidney has its own artery (to take blood to it), vein (to take blood from it) and ureter (to take urine to the bladder).

The artery belonging to the new kidney is attached to the patient's main artery supplying blood to the leg on that side of the body. The vein belonging to the new kidney is attached to the main vein carrying blood from that leg. These leg blood vessels are big enough to be able to send blood to and from the new kidney without affecting the blood supply to the leg. The transplant kidney's ureter is attached to the patient's own bladder. A small plastic pipe (called a double J stent) is usually inserted into the ureter (see *diagram 3*) to help prevent the ureter from becoming blocked after the operation. At the end of the operation, the patient's abdomen is closed with stitches.

POST-OPERATIVE TUBES

When the patient wakes up from the anaesthetic, they will have several tubes coming out of them. These will include:

- a urinary catheter (a tube into the bladder);
- a central venous pressure (CVP) line (which is placed under the collarbone or in the side of the neck, and measures the pressure of blood inside the heart);
- an intravenous drip in the arm (to give the patient fluid and drugs if necessary); and, probably,
- one or more surgical drains coming out of the abdomen (to drain off any fluid that gathers around the kidney after the operation).

These tubes will be removed one by one over the next few days. The urinary catheter is usually left in place for five days or more. The double J stent is usually removed during a small operation (under local or general anaesthetic) about three months after the transplant. PD patients will also have their PD catheter removed at the same time. Some haemodialysis patients find that their fistula stops working at some stage after the transplant. This does not matter, provided that the transplant is working well.

AFTER THE OPERATION

The first few days after the operation are critical and patients are monitored very closely. Particular attention is paid to blood pressure, fluid intake and urine output. Most patients are able to drink and eat small amounts and also to sit out of bed the day after the operation.

Patients will have their blood creatinine level measured every day. This shows whether or not the transplant kidney is working. The amount of urine that the new kidney makes is not a reliable indicator, as people who have just had a transplant may produce a large volume of urine that does not contain many toxins.

Transplant operation

1 Incision sites (see Note below)
2 New kidney position (right side insertion)
3 Double J stent tube (shown in position)

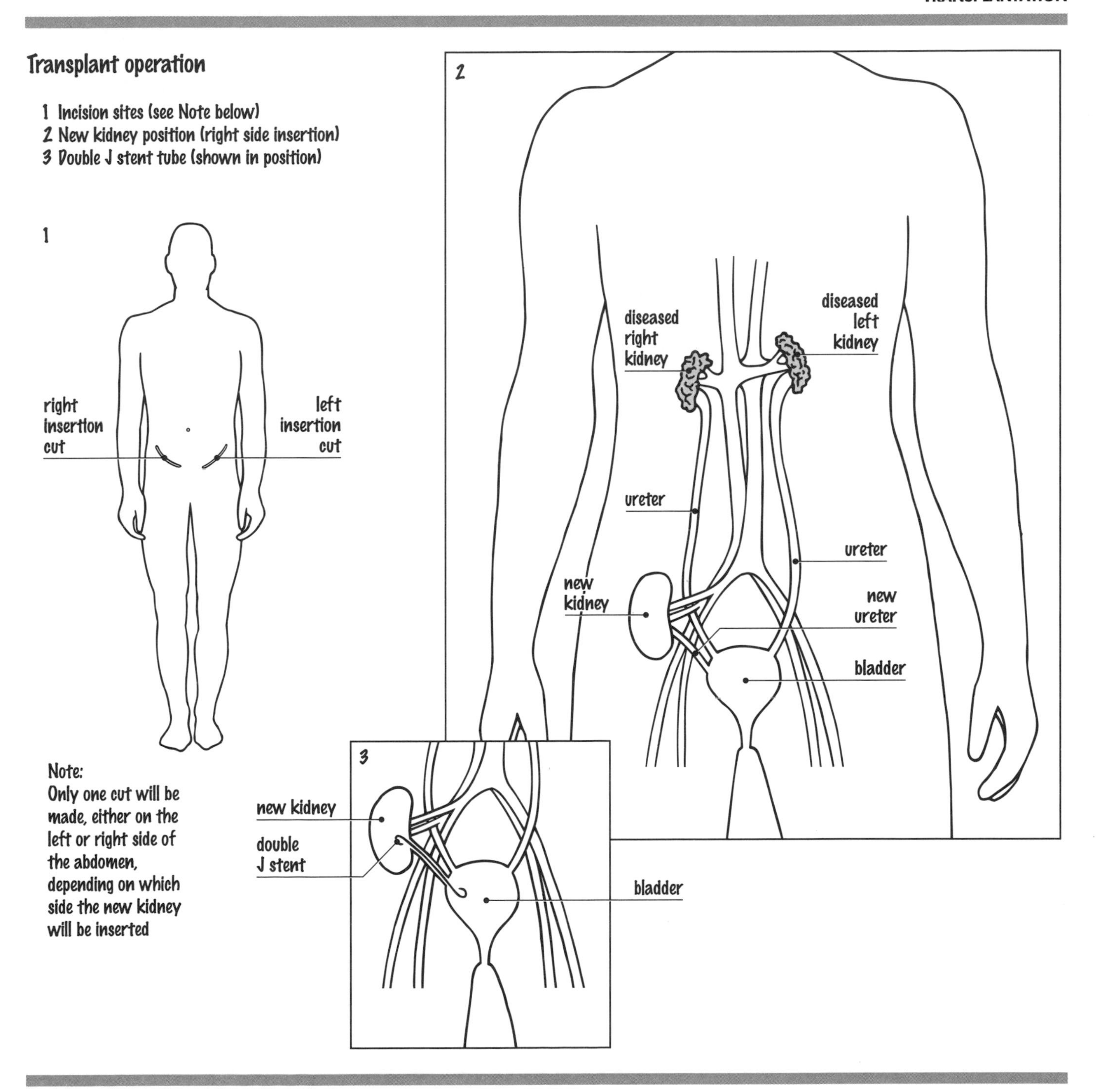

Note:
Only one cut will be made, either on the left or right side of the abdomen, depending on which side the new kidney will be inserted

In about one third of kidney transplant patients, the kidney does not produce any urine in the first few days (and sometimes weeks) after the transplant. This does not mean that the transplant will never work. If the transplant does not work at the start, patients will need to continue dialysis and play a waiting game until the kidney starts working. A 'good transplant' is one that is working well after one year, not two weeks.

Patients will usually stay in hospital for about two weeks. After leaving hospital, they will need to go to clinic very frequently for many months – initially two or three times per week, then once a week, then once every two weeks, etc. When the doctors are satisfied that the kidney is working well, the patient's appointments may be extended to once every three months or so.

It usually takes three to six months for patients who have had a kidney transplant to return to normal activities, including work. Transplant patients are recommended not to drive for at least one month after the operation. The function of the kidney, and the risk of infection, will not be affected by having sex. However, it is probably best not to resume sexual activity until about four weeks after leaving hospital.

How long will the transplant last?

A kidney transplant does not last for ever. The average life-span of a transplanted kidney is eight years for a cadaveric kidney, and about 11 years for a living related transplant. The average for a living unrelated transplant is somewhere between the two. So, the 'best' (longest lasting) kidney transplant is one from a relative, then a friend or partner, then a dead person.

Another way of looking at how long a transplanted kidney is likely to last is to look at the percentage chance that the kidney will be working at set time points.

A transplanted cadaveric kidney has, on average:

- an 80–90% chance of working one year after the operation;
- a 60% chance of lasting five years;
- a 50% chances of lasting ten years or more.

The chances that a kidney from a non-heart-beating donor will still be working at the same time points are about 10% worse than this. The chances that a kidney donated by a living person will be working at these times are about 10% better.

So, younger patients may need two or more transplants in their lives. If a transplant fails, the patient can restart dialysis, and go back on the transplant waiting list.

Possible problems after a transplant

Although a transplant is an excellent treatment for most people with ESRF, it is not problem-free. Most people who have had a transplant experience a problem called rejection (see *below* for details). Rejection is part of the reason why transplants do not last for ever.

Other problems that a patient may experience after a transplant are drug side effects (see *page 68*), infection (see *page 69*) and cancer (see *page 70*). It must also be said that within one year of any transplant a small percentage of patients die. However, this percentage is no greater than the percentage of patients with ESRF that would have died if they had remained on dialysis.

The rejection process

'Rejection' means that the patient's body recognises that the transplanted kidney is not 'its own' and tries to 'reject' it from the body. Even when patients and transplant kidneys are apparently 'well-matched' (in terms of blood group and tissue type, see *pages 59-60*), some degree of rejection is common. The severity of rejection varies from patient to patient. Rejection may be either acute (see *below*) or chronic (see *page 68*).

The body system that is responsible for the rejection process is called the immune system. The immune system is the body's natural defence system. It is located all over the body, and has many different parts. It includes organs (such as the spleen and appendix), lymph nodes (including the 'glands' in the neck) and specialist white blood cells (called lymphocytes).

The usual task of the immune system is to fight foreign invaders. These include germs (such as bacteria and viruses) and foreign objects (such as splinters or thorns embedded in the skin). The immune system also fights cancer. An individual's immune system does not usually attack that person's own cells because these all have a 'friendly face' (consisting of special proteins called antigens on the outer surface of the cells). The immune system recognises the friendly face and knows to leave the cells alone. Germs and foreign objects do not have this friendly face. Nor do cancer cells, which have developed in an abnormal way.

Normally, the immune system is a 'good thing', as it protects the body from dangerous infections, foreign bodies and cancer. However, after a transplant it can be a 'bad thing'. If the immune system recognises that the new kidney does not have the usual friendly face of the body's own cells, it will become overactive and send lymphocytes to attack (reject) the kidney. The body is actually trying to protect you from the kidney, which it perceives as a danger. Luckily, there are drugs – called immuno-suppressant drugs (see *page 68*) – that can help prevent and treat the rejection process.

ACUTE REJECTION

'Acute' means short-term and of rapid onset, requiring immediate action. Acute rejection can occur in the first few months (particularly the first few weeks) after a transplant. It is very common – about 40% of patients experience acute rejection in the first three months after a transplant. If acute rejection hasn't occurred within one year of the operation, then it is unlikely to happen.

Acute rejection may sometimes cause pain and fever, but usually there are no symptoms. Doctors will suspect that a patient has acute rejection if the blood creatinine is either not coming down after a transplant, or if it has started to fall and then remains stable or increases again. However, acute rejection is not the only reason why there may be problems with blood creatinine levels after a transplant, and these other possibilities are usually looked for first.

Investigation. Tests that might be performed include an ultrasound scan (a sound-wave picture). This will show if the patient's ureter (the tube that takes urine from the kidney to the bladder) is blocked. Other possibilities are specialist scanning techniques called a radio-isotope scan and a Doppler scan. Either of these will show if there are any problems with the blood supply to the new kidney.

The only way to be sure whether a transplant kidney is being rejected is to do a test called a biopsy. For this test, a hollow needle called a biopsy needle is used to remove a very small piece of the new kidney. This piece of kidney is then looked at very carefully under a microscope for any signs of rejection. It is common for patients who have had a kidney transplant to have two or more biopsies in the weeks after the operation.

Treatment. If the biopsy shows signs of rejection, then the patient will be given a high-dose steroid drug called *methylprednisolone*. This drug will be given by intravenous injection, once a day for three days. These are called 'pulses' of *methylprednisolone*. Very often, this treatment will suppress the rejection process, and the creatinine will start to decrease. Occasionally, a patient may need two courses of this drug.

If pulse *methylprednisolone* does not work, the patient may be given a five- to ten-day course of a stronger intravenous injection, such as *anti-lymphocyte globulin (ALG), anti-thymocyte globulin (ATG) or orthoclone K T-cell receptor 3 (OKT3) antibody*. These almost always work and the rejection process goes away. However, all of them can have fairly severe side effects; especially OKT3, which can cause fever, diarrhoea, joint and muscle pain, wheeze, and shortness of breath due to fluid on the lungs (pulmonary oedema).

CHRONIC REJECTION

'Chronic' means long-term and of slow onset, not necessarily requiring prompt action. Some doctors think that the term 'chronic rejection' is misleading. The condition it describes is very different from acute rejection. In chronic rejection, there is no true rejection process taking place. The patient's immune system does not attack and reject the transplant kidney.

Chronic rejection is more like a slow ageing of the new kidney. The cause is uncertain. If it happens, it will usually be more than a year after the transplant operation. Doctors may suspect chronic rejection if a patient's blood creatinine starts to rise slowly after it has been stable for some time. As with acute rejection (see *above*), the only sure way to diagnose the condition is to do a biopsy. There is no treatment for chronic rejection.

The severity of chronic rejection varies. Mild chronic rejection is not usually a problem. However, more severe chronic rejection will eventually lead to failure of the kidney (and therefore to restarting dialysis or having another transplant). Chronic rejection may take years to happen, but it is much the most common cause of transplant failure after the first year.

IMMUNO-SUPPRESSANT DRUGS

All patients who have a kidney transplant need to take drugs called immuno-suppressant drugs. As the name immuno-suppressant suggests, the function of these drugs is to suppress the immune system. The aim is to dampen down the immune system sufficiently to stop it rejecting the transplant kidney, while still keeping it active enough to fight infection. Finding the balance can be quite difficult.

The most commonly used immuno-suppressants are currently *cyclosporin*, *azathioprine* and *prednisolone* (a steroid); but newer drugs, such as *tacrolimus* (*FK506*, often called *'FK'*, an alternative to *cyclosporin*) and *mycophenylate* (an alternative to *azathoprine*), are also becoming available.

Although transplant patients will no longer usually need to continue taking EPO or calcium tablets, it is vital for them to take two or three different kinds of immuno-suppressant drugs every day. This is because if they stop taking the drugs, the immune system 'fights back'. If a patient is unable to take their immuno-suppressant drugs, either because they have run out or because they are suffering from diarrhoea or vomiting, they should go to the hospital at once. The immune system does not forget that there is a 'foreign' kidney in the body. It is always waiting for a chance to attack and reject it.

DRUG SIDE EFFECTS

All three of the most commonly used immuno-suppressant drugs have their problems:

Cyclosporin. This is the most important drug used to prevent kidney rejection. Unfortunately, if patients are given too much of it, *cyclosporin* is itself toxic to the kidney, and can prevent the transplant from working. This condition is called *cyclosporin* toxicity. *Cyclosporin* can also damage the liver. To reduce the risk of problems, patients on *cyclosporin* will have the amount of the drug in their blood monitored regularly. If problems do occur, these can usually be reversed either by stopping the drug or reducing the dose.

Some patients who take *cyclosporin* for a long time develop a condition called gum hypertrophy. This is an excessive growth of the gums, which can be unsightly. It is less likely to develop if patients practise good dental hygiene, including regular flossing between the teeth. Another possible side effect of *cyclosporin* is excessive growth of hair on the face and body.

If the side effects of *cyclosporin* are severe, *tacrolimus* may be used in its place.

Azathioprine. The main problem with *azathioprine* is that it can suppress activity in the bone marrow, where blood cells are made. By affecting blood cell production, *azathioprine* can cause a number of serious problems. If too few red blood cells are produced, the patient will suffer from anaemia, causing tiredness. If there are too few white blood cells, the patient will develop a condition called neutropenia. This lack of white blood cells will affect the patient's ability to fight infection. If too few of the blood cells called platelets are produced, the resulting problem is thrombocytopenia, which can cause an increased tendency to bleed.

Patients taking *azathioprine* may suffer from any or all of the above problems. However, stopping the drug or reducing the dose will normally put matters right. *Azathioprine* can also damage the liver.

Prednisolone. This drug is a steroid and, like other steroid drugs, it can cause thinning of the skin (leading to easy bruising), and facial swelling (giving a red and rounded appearance to the face). These problems may lessen if the dose of the drug is reduced.

Taking *prednisolone* can also cause diabetes mellitus ('sugar diabetes'). At worst, this might mean that the patient will have to take tablets or give themselves *insulin* injections.

A further possible problem with *prednisolone* is that it can cause bone weakness, which may in the long-term lead to crumbling of the joints, especially the hip joints. Replacement of one or both hips may become necessary.

INFECTION

Although immuno-suppressant drugs help prevent transplant rejection by making the immune system less efficient, their effect on a patient's ability to fight infections is generally less than might be expected. So, most people taking immuno-suppressant drugs do not get infection after infection.

Having said that, there is one infection that is a particular problem after transplantation. It is called cytomegalovirus (CMV). For most people who are not taking immuno-suppressant drugs, CMV is a mild infection that causes a 'flu-like illness. However, in patients who have just received a transplant, CMV infection can be quite a severe illness.

If a transplant patient does ever get the virus, there is a very effective treatment for it. This is called *gancyclovir*, and is given as a course of injections.

CANCER

One of the functions of the immune system is to fight cancer. By making the immune system less efficient to help prevent transplant rejection, immuno-suppressant drugs unfortunately increase the likelihood of getting some types of cancer. A research study has shown that 25% of transplant patients who live for 25 years after a transplant develop some type of cancer.

Transplant patients are three times more likely than other people to get skin cancers after a transplant. This makes it very important for people who have had a transplant to use a strong 'sun block' cream to avoid sunburn. Exposure to the sun greatly increases the risk of developing skin cancer. (In Australia, where skin cancer is particularly common, the increased risk to transplant patients rises to 40 times the average.) Provided that skin cancers are diagnosed in good time, they are not usually a major problem. This type of cancer does not usually spread to other parts of the body, and can be easily removed.

A small number (1-2%) of transplant patients develop a more serious cancer called lymphoma, usually within a year of the operation. This cancer affects cells in the body's immune system (mainly in the spleen and lymph nodes). Most people who develop lymphoma after a transplant die within two years of the diagnosis.

KEY FACTS

1. For the right patient at the right time, a transplant is the best treatment for ESRF.
2. If a transplant works well, the patient will be totally free from dialysis.
3. Many patients with kidney failure are suitable for a transplant. Suitability for a transplant is more important than age.
4. Transplants are matched to the patient in terms of blood group and tissue type.
5. Transplant kidneys come from three sources: cadaveric transplants, living related transplants and living unrelated transplants.
6. The transplant waiting list works on the basis of finding the 'right' kidney for the 'right' person – i.e., patients do not join a queue.
7. Patients have to wait on the transplant waiting list for an average of about two years.
8. A transplant operation lasts two to three hours and involves staying in hospital for about two weeks after the operation.
9. A transplant does not last for ever. Transplants from living relatives last longest.
10. If a transplant fails, the patient can go back to dialysis or have another transplant.
11. Patients have to take immuno-suppressant drugs daily to prevent their body rejecting a transplant. These drugs have side effects.
12. Transplant patients have an increased risk of developing some types of cancer.

11 BLOOD TESTS

The information in this chapter will help people with kidney failure to understand their own blood test results.

INTRODUCTION

All patients with kidney failure have regular blood tests. This chapter is mainly written for patients on dialysis, but the general principles described here are also true for patients who have not yet started dialysis or who have had a kidney transplant. Blood test results provide doctors and nurses with the information they need to treat their kidney patients as effectively as possible. Patients who learn to read their own blood test results can find out a lot about what is going on inside their body. They can also assess for themselves how well their treatment is working.

THE 'FIGURES'

The term 'figures' is commonly used in hospitals to refer to the biochemistry blood test that most kidney patients have at the end of every clinic appointment.

The biochemistry blood test is not really a single test. It includes measurements of a whole range of different substances in the blood. Most patients with kidney failure tend to focus on two of them: creatinine and potassium. This is a good choice, as they are probably the two most important tests. Both of them indicate how well dialysis is working.

However, looking at your blood test results can tell you a lot more about your body. They can tell you about the levels of minerals in the body, the acidity of the blood, the state of your bones, how well nourished you are, and how well your liver is working.

The dozen or so substances usually measured in a biochemistry blood test for kidney patients can be divided into two groups: dialysable and non-dialysable. Dialysable substances are ones that can be removed from, or added to, the body during dialysis. Non-dialysable substances are ones that cannot be removed from, or added to, the body during dialysis.

TESTS FOR DIALYSABLE SUBSTANCES

The first group of substances measured in the biochemistry blood test for kidney patients are all dialysable. This means that they can pass from the blood into the dialysis solution, and vice versa. The direction in which a dialysable substance travels during dialysis depends on the amount of substance in the blood and in the dialysis solution. Substances always pass – by a process called diffusion – from a stronger to a weaker solution. (See *Chapter 7* for a more detailed description of this basic principle of dialysis.)

By putting more or less of different substances in the dialysis fluid, as compared to the blood, it is possible to remove substances from the blood, or to add them to the body. The biochemistry test measures blood levels of several substances that may be removed from the body by dialysis – potassium, creatinine, urea and phosphate. It also measures the levels of some useful substances that are given to patients in the dialysis fluid – bicarbonate and calcium. Two other dialysable substances – sodium and glucose – are also measured, although blood levels of these substances are not usually affected by dialysis.

SODIUM

Sodium is one of the minerals normally present in the blood. Its name is sometimes written as 'Na' (pronounced 'N'...'a'), which is the chemical symbol for sodium. The normal level of sodium in the blood is 135–145 mmol/l (millimoles per litre of blood). Sodium keeps water in the body, and helps to control the blood pressure.

Sodium levels are not usually a problem for people with kidney failure. However, sodium is a dialysable substance. To keep blood levels normal, it is therefore necessary to prevent it from being lost from the blood into the dialysis fluid. This is done by having a similar concentration of sodium in the dialysis fluid to that in the blood. (PD fluid contains 132 mmol/l of sodium; haemodialysis fluid contains 132–145 mmol/l.) Because the levels of sodium in the dialysis fluid and the blood are similar, dialysis does not have much effect on the blood sodium level.

Controlling the level of sodium in the blood is quite easy when someone is on dialysis. A normal level is usually achieved.

POTASSIUM

Potassium is another dialysable mineral that is normally present in the blood. The chemical symbol for potassium is 'K'. The normal level of potassium in the blood is 3.5–5.0 mmol/l. Potassium helps the heart to function properly.

Patients with kidney failure tend to have too much potassium in the blood, although there are some patients who have too little. Either too much or too little potassium can be dangerous, causing the heart to stop and the patient to die. Problems are especially likely if the blood potassium is more than 7.0 mmol/l, or less than 2.0 mmol/l.

There is no potassium in PD dialysis fluid, and only a small amount (usually less than 2.0 mmol/l) in haemodialysis fluid. Because of the basic principle of dialysis (by which substances pass from a stronger to a weaker solution), potassium therefore usually flows out of the blood into the dialysis fluid. Dialysis therefore normally removes potassium from the body.

Controlling the level of potassium in the blood can be quite difficult, especially in patients who are being treated by haemodialysis. Because of this, it may be necessary for haemodialysis patients to restrict their intake of potassium-rich foods (see also *Chapter 12, page 83*). Despite the difficulties, a normal potassium level can usually be achieved.

GLUCOSE

The normal level of glucose in the blood is 3.0–7.8 mmol/l. Glucose is a type of sugar, and it provides the body with energy. The amount of glucose in the blood is controlled by a substance called insulin, which is made in the pancreas (a gland in the upper abdomen). When someone has diabetes mellitus ('sugar diabetes'), their pancreas makes either no insulin, or not enough, and their blood glucose tends to be high.

Blood glucose levels are only usually a problem for the 40% or so of patients with kidney failure who also have diabetes. Blood glucose problems in these patients are due to the diabetes itself, rather than to the kidney failure that was caused by the diabetes.

For kidney patients who do not have diabetes, it is usually easy to achieve a normal blood glucose level. So blood glucose is not something that most dialysis patients have to worry about.

Although glucose is a dialysable substance, it does not do what people might expect it to do during dialysis. First, for haemodialysis, the dialysis fluid contains a similar amount of glucose to that in the blood (about 5 mmol/l). As expected, given the basic principle of dialysis, very little glucose passes between the blood and the dialysis fluid.

Second, the dialysis fluid used for PD contains a lot of glucose. Even a weak bag contains about 75.5 mmol/l (which is more than ten times the normal blood level of glucose). In this case, it might be assumed that glucose would pour into the patient and cause problems. In fact, the body quickly deals with the sudden inflow of glucose. As soon the glucose enters the bloodstream, the pancreas can usually produce enough insulin to bring the level of glucose in the blood back down to normal.

However, if a PD patient uses a lot of 'strong' bags (containing 3.86% glucose, compared to 1.36% in weak bags), the amount of glucose entering the blood may be too much for the pancreas to cope with. This extra glucose may make any patient (diabetic or not) put on body weight, usually as fat. If a patient has diabetes, it may also upset diabetic control, making it necessary to inject more insulin, or to take more tablets.

Given that glucose sometimes causes problems for PD patients, you may wonder if it is really necessary to include it in the dialysis fluid. In fact, the glucose in the PD fluid is there to perform one of the two major tasks of the kidney, i.e., to remove water from the body.

Creatinine

Creatinine is a waste substance produced by the muscles whenever they are used. Like thousands of other body wastes, creatinine is carried around the body in the blood until it is normally filtered out by the kidneys and passed in the urine (see *page 1*).

Creatinine is not itself harmful to the body, but it is a very important 'marker', which provides a valuable guide to the levels of other, less easily measured substances in the blood. If there is a build-up of creatinine in the blood, there will also be a build-up of many other more harmful substances. The higher the creatinine level, the worse is the kidney, dialysis or transplant function (see *Chapter 2* for more details).

The normal level of creatinine in the blood is 45–120 µmol/l (micromoles per litre of blood). There is no creatinine in dialysis fluid. Because creatinine is dialysable, it will therefore pass out of the blood, through the dialysis membrane, into the dialysis fluid.

Creatinine levels can never be normal when someone is on dialysis. Dialysis – PD or haemodialysis – can provide only about 5% of the function of two healthy kidneys.

For a patient of average size who is on PD, the target creatinine level is below 800 µmol/l. For a similar patient on haemodialysis, the target is below 800 μmol/l before dialysis, and below 300 μmol/l after dialysis. Because larger, more muscular people produce more creatinine than smaller, less muscular people, individual creatinine targets are adjusted to take account of body and muscle size. Provided this adjustment is made, the creatinine level is a very reliable guide to a patient's kidney (dialysis or transplant) function (see *Chapter 2* for more details).

UREA

Urea is a waste product of food. It is made in the liver and then travels in the blood to the kidneys, where it normally goes into the urine for removal from the body. Like creatinine, urea is a 'marker' for other more harmful substances in the blood. A build-up of urea in the blood also indicates a build-up of many other substances. The higher the blood urea level, the worse is the kidney, dialysis or transplant function (see *Chapter 2* for more details).

The normal range for urea in the blood is 3.3–6.7 mmol/l. There is no urea in dialysis fluid. Again, because urea is dialysable, it will pass out of the blood into the dialysis fluid. Urea levels can never be normal when someone is on dialysis. Neither type of dialysis is good enough at getting rid of it. For patients on PD, the usual target level for urea is below 25 mmol/l. For haemodialysis patients, the usual targets are below 25 mmol/l before dialysis and below 9 mmol/l after dialysis.

Blood urea levels provide a less reliable guide than blood creatinine levels to a patient's kidney, dialysis or transplant function. This is because the amount of urea in the blood is also affected by what a patient eats and by how much fluid there is in the body.

BICARBONATE

The normal level of bicarbonate in the blood is 22–30 mmol/l. If the blood bicarbonate is lower than normal, this means that there is too much acid in the blood. Acid is a waste product of food, which, like other wastes in the blood, is normally removed by the kidneys. When someone has kidney failure, the level of acid in the blood goes up and the level of bicarbonate falls. If acid levels in the blood are not adequately corrected over a period of time, this may contribute to malnutrition (loss of flesh weight, see *Chapter 12, page 81* for more information). Malnutrition is a common problem in dialysis patients.

The target level for bicarbonate is normal, preferably high normal, say 26 mmol/l or over. For haemodialysis patients, the target applies after dialysis. It does not matter if the bicarbonate is consistently above normal.

In order to keep the acidity of the blood normal, dialysis fluid contains an alkali (a substance that is the opposite of an acid). In haemodialysis fluid, the alkali is either bicarbonate (at a concentration of 35 mmol/l) or acetate (at a concentration of 40 mmol/l). In PD fluid, the alkali is lactate, at a concentration of either 35 or 40 mmol/l. Both acetate and lactate are changed into bicarbonate (the body's natural alkali) inside the body.

The level of alkali in the dialysis fluid is higher than the level of alkali in the blood. Because alkali is dialysable, and because of the basic principle of dialysis, alkali passes from the dialysis fluid into the patient. In the blood, the alkali neutralises the acid and produces normal blood bicarbonate levels.

CALCIUM

Calcium is a mineral that strengthens the bones. One of the functions of the kidneys is to help to keep calcium in the bones. When someone has kidney failure, calcium passes out of the bones. There is also a fall in the level of calcium in the blood. (See *Chapter 6* for more information about calcium and the bones.)

The normal level of calcium in the blood is 2.2–2.6 mmol/l. Calcium is a dialysable substance. This means that it can be given to kidney patients in the dialysis fluid. If there is a higher concentration of calcium in the dialysis fluid than there is in the blood, calcium will pass into the patient's blood during dialysis.

The level of calcium in dialysis fluid ranges from 2.0 mmol/l to 3.5 mmol/l. Different doctors prefer different levels of calcium in the dialysis fluid – all have their advantages. Most dialysis fluids allow calcium to flow into the blood.

The target level for calcium is 2.5–2.6 mmol/l. This level, at the top of the normal range, has been found to be better for kidney patients than calcium levels in the middle of the range.

If the dialysis fluid does not give a patient enough calcium to achieve the target level, it may be necessary to take calcium carbonate tablets (as *Calcichew*, for example) or vitamin D tablets (usually as *alfacalcidol*).

PHOSPHATE

The normal level of phosphate in the blood is 0.8–1.4 mmol/l. In normal quantities, phosphate helps calcium to strengthen the bones. Healthy kidneys help to keep the right amount of phosphate in the blood. When someone has kidney failure, the level of phosphate in the blood rises. (See *Chapter 6* for more information about phosphate and the bones.)

Phosphate is a dialysable substance and the aim is to reduce the amount of phosphate in the blood of people with kidney failure. This is the reason that there is no phosphate in dialysis fluid. Phosphate therefore passes from the patient's blood into the dialysis fluid (because of the basic principle of dialysis, by which substances pass from a stronger to a weaker solution).

The target phosphate level for dialysis patients is less than 1.8 mmol/l. It is not usually possible to achieve normal phosphate levels in dialysis patients. Dialysis is simply not good enough at removing phosphate from the blood.

If dialysis does not keep blood phosphate at the target level, it may be necessary to take calcium carbonate tablets (as *Calcichew*, for example). Not only do these tablets give calcium to a patient, they also reduce the level of phosphate in the blood.

TESTS FOR NON-DIALYSABLE SUBSTANCES

The next group of blood tests to be looked at in this chapter are those that measure blood levels of various non-dialysable substances. Like the tests already described, these tests – measuring blood levels of albumin and various substances such as bilirubin that show liver function – form part of the regular biochemistry test for patients with kidney failure.

ALBUMIN

Albumin is a type of body protein. It is made in the liver and is present in the blood. The normal level of albumin in the blood is 35–50 g/l (grams per litre of blood).

The level of albumin in the blood is measured because of the information this provides about whether a patient is eating enough (especially enough protein). Kidney failure tends to reduce appetite. Also, during dialysis, some albumin and other proteins are lost into the dialysis fluid.

SUMMARY OF NORMAL AND TARGET BLOOD TEST RESULTS FOR PATIENTS ON DIALYSIS

Substance	Relevance	Normal level	Target level	Units
Dialysable substances				
Sodium	Fluid balance	135-145	normal	mmol/l
Potassium	Heart health	3.5-5.0	normal	mmol/l
Glucose	Blood sugar	3.0-7.8	normal	mmol/l
Creatinine	Toxin clearance	45-120	less than 800	µmol/l
Urea	Toxin clearance	3.3-6.7	less than 25	mmol/l
Bicarbonate	Acid balance	22-30	high-normal (26-30)	mmol/l
Calcium	Bone health	2.2-2.6	high-normal (2.5-2.6)	mmol/l
Phosphate	Bone health	0.8-1.4	less than 1.8	mmol/l
Non-dialysable substances				
Albumin	Nutritional status	35-50	normal	g/l
Bilirubin	Liver function	3-20	normal	mmol/l
AST	Liver function	10-50	normal	iu/l
Alk. phos.	Liver function	30-130	normal	iu/l
GammaGT	Liver function	5-55	normal	iu/l
Other (non-dialysable) substances				
Haemoglobin (man)	Blood health	13-16.5	10-12	g/dl
Haemoglobin (woman)	Blood health	11.5-15.5	10-12	g/dl
Ferritin (man)	Iron in blood	15-300	more than 200	µg/l
Ferritin (woman)	Iron in blood	10-200	more than 200	µg/l
Parathyroid hormone	Bone health	(variable)	less than 3 x upper limit of normal	(variable)

How do your test results compare? Although your hospital may use slightly different figures, they should be similar to those given here. If any of your figures do not seem to be on target, find out why.

Many kidney patients have lower than normal blood albumin levels. If a patient's blood albumin level is always low, malnutrition (loss of flesh weight, see *Chapter 12, page 81*) may have become a problem.

Unfortunately, the information obtained by measuring blood albumin levels is not very reliable. One difficulty is that the blood albumin decreases very quickly whenever someone is ill. This means that it is not possible to tell whether the malnutrition diagnosed by the test is really a long-term problem or not. Another problem with the test is that the blood albumin tends to fall whatever is wrong with a patient, no matter how well nourished they are. A further problem with this test is that even if a fall in the blood albumin level is identified, there are no specific treatments to bring it back up again. The target level, for what it is worth, is normal.

Liver function tests

The results of a group of tests called liver function tests (LFTs) often appear at the bottom of biochemistry test results. Most doctors do not mention these, or brush over them, saying 'Oh, don't worry about them, they are just liver tests'. So, why are they measured? The main reason is that biochemistry tests are generally done by a machine, which includes the liver tests automatically.

Having said that, patients with kidney failure can get liver problems. Haemodialysis, blood transfusions or a kidney transplant put patients at increased risk of catching a viral infection that can cause liver failure. Also, some of the drugs that are used to suppress the immune system after a kidney transplant can affect the liver. So, here is a quick guide to common LFTs:

- **Bilirubin.** This is the most important of the LFTs. (It is the liver function equivalent of the creatinine test.) Bilirubin is produced when worn out red blood cells are broken down for removal from the body. The normal range of levels for bilirubin in the blood is 3–20 µmol/l (micromoles per litre of blood). Raised bilirubin levels show that the liver is not working properly. If the blood bilirubin goes above 50 µmol/l, the patient will develop jaundice (go yellow in colour).

- **Aspartate transaminase.** The normal range for aspartate transaminase (AST) in the blood is 10–50 iu/l (international units per litre). Raised levels indicate that liver cells have been damaged by disease.

- **Alkaline phosphatase.** The normal range for alkaline phosphatase (alk. phos.) in the blood is 30-130 iu/l. This test measures how well bile (a liquid made by the liver) drains from the liver. Bile contains the waste products from the liver. It is drained into the bowel, and leaves the body in the faeces. In dialysis patients, a high alk. phos. level usually indicates renal bone disease.

- **Gamma-glutamyltransferase.** The normal range for gamma-glutamyltransferase (GammaGT) in the blood is 5-55 iu/l. Like alkaline phosphatase measurements, this test measures how well bile drains from the liver.

Other blood tests

Kidney patients are also given a number of other blood tests in addition to the tests that make up their usual biochemistry test. The substances measured by these tests – haemoglobin, ferritin and parathyroid hormone – are all non-dialysable. Kidney patients have their haemoglobin levels measured each time they have a biochemistry blood test. Their blood levels of ferritin and parathyroid hormone are measured less often, usually every six months or so.

HAEMOGLOBIN

Most patients on dialysis have anaemia. Anaemia means that there is not enough of a substance called haemoglobin in the blood. Haemoglobin is important because it carries oxygen around the body. Every part of the body needs a regular supply of oxygen. (See *Chapter 5* for more information about anaemia in kidney patients.)

Haemoglobin levels in the blood are measured by a test called a haemoglobin or Hb. The normal level of Hb is 11.5–15.5 g/dl (grams per decilitre of blood) in a woman, and 13–16.5 g/dl in a man. If the Hb level is below 11.5 g/dl in a woman, and below 13 g/dl in a man, the patient is said to be anaemic.

There is a very good treatment for anaemia called erythropoietin (EPO), which is given as an injection 1–3 times per week. Dialysis patients who are not being treated with EPO may have an Hb of only 6–8 g/dl, which is very low. The aim of EPO treatment is to increase the Hb level to 10-12 g/dl. (See *Chapter 5* for more information on EPO.)

FERRITIN

For EPO (see *above*) to work well, it is necessary to have enough iron in the body. The best guide to how much iron there is in the body is a blood test that measures the level of a substance called ferritin. The more iron there is in the body, the higher the level of ferritin in the blood.

To help EPO to work, it is important to have a ferritin level of at least 200 mg/l (milligrams per litre of blood). As with Hb levels (see *above*), the normal level of ferritin is different in men (15-300 mg/l) and women (10-200 mg/l). Nonetheless, 200 mg/l is an adequate level in both sexes.

To keep the ferritin above 200 mg/l, many patients on EPO have to take iron tablets, or to have regular iron injections . Some renal units now give iron injections to all patients with kidney failure, whether they are on EPO or not.

PARATHYROID HORMONE

Parathyroid hormone (PTH) is a hormone (a chemical messenger) that is made by four glands in the front of the neck. These glands are too small to see or feel. If someone with kidney failure has low levels of calcium and/or high levels of phosphate for a long time, these glands grow and start producing too much PTH.

It is important to measure the level of PTH in the blood of patients with kidney failure because of the information this test provides about a patient's bones. The amount of PTH in the blood is the best long-term guide to how much damage kidney failure has done to the bones. Blood levels of calcium and phosphate tell you what is happening now, PTH also tells you what will happen in the future.

Different renal units use different tests for measuring PTH, and different doctors have different views about PTH targets for kidney patients. A PTH level that is less than three times the upper limit of normal is generally considered to be satisfactory. As with phosphate levels, it is often hard to achieve normal PTH levels in people with kidney failure. (See *Chapter 6* for more information about PTH and renal bone disease.)

KEY FACTS

1. The term 'figures' is used to refer to the biochemistry blood test that most kidney patients have at the end of every clinic appointment.
2. The biochemistry test is not a single blood test. It measures the levels of a dozen or so different substances in the blood. The results tell you about the levels of minerals in the body, the acidity of the blood, the state of your bones, how well nourished you are, and how well your liver is working.
3. The substances that are measured can be divided into two groups: dialysable and non-dialysable.
4. Dialysable substances can pass from the blood into the dialysis fluid, and vice versa. Substances pass from a stronger to a weaker solution. This basic principle of dialysis determines the direction in which a substance travels during dialysis.
5. Potassium, creatinine, urea and phosphate are dialysable substances that are taken out of the body during dialysis.
6. Calcium and bicarbonate are dialysable substances that are put into the body during dialysis.
7. Non-dialysable substances measured by blood tests include albumin, various substances that measure liver function, haemoglobin, ferritin and parathyroid hormone.

12 DIET

This chapter explains why it is important for people with kidney failure to watch what they eat. It also describes the different dietary advice that they are likely to be given as their condition and treatment change.

INTRODUCTION

One of the questions most frequently asked by kidney patients is, 'Why does the advice given to me about my diet keep changing?' Well, it isn't because the dietitian got it wrong in the first place! The reason is that patients' dietary needs change as their condition changes. So, just as drug therapy and other treatments may need to be altered, so diet may need to be revised to stay in line.

'HEALTHY EATING GUIDELINES'

It is a good idea for all patients with kidney failure – whether pre-dialysis, on dialysis, or with a transplant – to follow 'Healthy Eating Guidelines'.

These guidelines are:

- to eat some high-fibre foods (such as wholemeal bread and cereals);
- to eat only moderate amounts of fats (which should be mainly polyunsaturated);
- to avoid adding 'extra' salt to foods if you have high blood pressure.

WHAT IS 'NUTRITIONAL STATUS'?

The term 'nutritional status' is used by doctors, nurses and dietitians to describe a patient's state of nourishment. A person with a poor nutritional status is not receiving enough of the right kinds of food.

There is no single reliable method of measuring nutritional status. There is no nutritional equivalent of the blood creatinine test (see *Chapter 2*).

Doctors, nurses or dietitians usually assess the nutritional status of a kidney patient by:

- asking how the patient is feeling;
- asking about the patient's diet (perhaps including asking the patient to keep a record for a while of everything they eat and drink);
- measuring the level of albumin (a type of protein) in the blood (see *page 77*);
- measuring the size of the patient's muscles;
- monitoring the patient's body weight.

Research has shown that nutritional status is an important factor in survival. One recent study of 12,000 haemodialysis patients in the USA showed that patients who had a very low blood albumin when they started dialysis were 17 times more likely to die in the first year of dialysis.

DIETARY PROTEIN AND KIDNEY FAILURE

Protein is an essential nutrient, which enables the body to build muscles, and to repair itself. The main sources of protein in the diet are meat, fish, dairy products and pulses (such as beans and lentils). Everyone – including people with kidney failure – must eat appropriate amounts of protein if they are to avoid serious nutritional problems.

When protein is digested, waste products are formed and enter the blood. One of these wastes is called urea (see *page 10*). Normal healthy kidneys are quite good at getting rid of urea and other wastes from the blood. However, as kidney failure develops, the kidneys become less and less able to remove wastes from the blood (see *Chapter 2*). Even so, this does not mean that people with kidney failure should stop eating protein (see *below*).

DIET BEFORE STARTING DIALYSIS

People with kidney failure who have not yet started dialysis should follow normal 'Healthy Eating Guidelines'. This includes continuing to eat foods that contain protein even after the level of urea in their blood has started to rise.

If people with kidney failure restrict their intake of dietary protein, their urea levels will not rise so rapidly. For this reason, it has been suggested that reducing the amount of protein in the diet might delay the need for dialysis. However, such use of protein restriction is controversial, since lower levels of urea in the blood may mean that patients are becoming malnourished – i.e., they are not receiving enough protein to maintain their flesh weight (see *page 16*).

When the time for dialysis draws closer, some patients do not feel as hungry as they used to – and some foods, particular meat products, may taste 'funny'. Special dietary supplements may help such patients to maintain adequate protein, energy and vitamin intakes. A dietitian will be able to provide advice about these supplements.

DIET DURING DIALYSIS

Several aspects of diet and nutrition are very important for patients on dialysis. All kidney patients are at an increased risk of developing malnutrition (see *below*).

It may also be necessary to pay special attention to a dialysis patient's intake of phosphate, calcium, potassium, salt, fluid and vitamins (see below, *pages 82-84*). In some cases, there may also be other specific individual dietary recommendations (see *page 84*).

MALNUTRITION AND KIDNEY FAILURE

The term malnutrition means severe loss of flesh weight, usually due to not eating enough (especially foods providing protein and energy). It is the most important, and most dangerous, nutritional problem that can develop in patients on either type of dialysis. So, to prevent malnutrition, patients on either type of dialysis will be asked to increase their food intake (especially their intake of protein).

Doctors are not entirely sure why kidney patients have an increased risk of malnutrition, and why they need extra protein in their diet. A combination of causes seems most likely.

POOR APPETITE AND MALNUTRITION

Probably the most important cause of malnutrition in kidney patients is the simplest one – poor appetite. This is one of the major symptoms of kidney failure, and is often the reason why people go to their family doctor in the first place.

When someone is pre-dialysis (or has a failing transplant), worsening of the appetite is one of the reasons why doctors start (or restart) dialysis. When a patient is on dialysis, a change – hopefully an improvement – in their appetite is often a more reliable guide to the effectiveness of the dialysis than are any of the blood tests (including the 'key' test, the blood creatinine, see *Chapter 2*).

Dialysis usually restores a kidney patient's appetite to near normal, though few dialysis patients ever really have a 'good' appetite. Dialysis is just not good enough at getting rid of the toxins that suppress appetite. (Doctors do not even know which these toxins are.)

If there is under-dialysis (i.e., a patient is not receiving enough dialysis), loss of appetite is one of the first symptoms of kidney failure to return. An increase in the dialysis dose will then probably help improve the patient's appetite. However, only a transplant will fully return a patient to a 'normal' appetite.

A build-up of toxins in the blood may not be the only reason for appetite problems in a kidney patient. Severe anaemia (see *Chapter 5*) may also suppress appetite.

Also, PD patients may have a poor appetite because of the dialysis fluid in their abdomen, which can make them feel bloated.

OTHER CAUSES OF MALNUTRITION

In addition to appetite problems, a number of other factors may contribute to the increased risk of malnutrition in kidney patients on dialysis.

PD patients lose protein and amino acids (substances from which proteins are built up) into their bags of dialysis fluid. Haemodialysis patients also lose amino acids into their dialysis fluid. So, kidney patients on both types of dialysis need extra protein in their diet to make up for these losses.

Infections also increase a person's requirements for high protein and high energy foods, and infections tend to be more common in dialysis patients.

A further possible cause of malnutrition in kidney patients is that some patients are not eating enough because of dietary restrictions imposed by their doctor or dietitian. (Fortunately, such over-zealous dietary restrictions are now going out of fashion.)

Loss of weight tends to be more common in haemodialysis than PD patients. PD patients have an extra source of calories – the sugar contained in PD fluid. Some of this is absorbed by the patient, providing the equivalent of approximately 300–500 calories a day – similar to eating between one and two Mars Bars. Haemodialysis patients don't have this extra energy source and may need additional dietary advice and supplements.

PROTEIN SUPPLEMENTS

Protein supplements can be very helpful if a kidney patient is not eating enough. These supplements are really very good and supply on average the equivalent protein of 2–3 oz of meat in 200 mls of fluid. The supplements are available on prescription, and hospital dietitians can ask their patients' GPs to prescribe them.

PHOSPHATE AND CALCIUM

Phosphate and calcium are two minerals that affect the health of the bones. When someone has kidney failure, the calcium levels in their body tend to be too low, and their phosphate levels too high. This puts them at risk of bone problems, due to a condition called renal bone disease (see *Chapter 6*).

Treatment for kidney patients therefore aims to raise blood calcium levels and also to lower blood phosphate levels. Both these aims can often be achieved by dialysis combined with taking calcium carbonate (e.g., *Calcichew*) tablets with meals, and sometimes by restricting phosphate in the diet.

A low phosphate diet is not as straightforward as it sounds. It is very difficult to cut down phosphate intake without also lowering protein intake.

Patients who need to adjust their diet to reduce their blood phosphate levels will be given specific advice by their dietitian. This will probably include asking them to be careful about eating dairy produce, offal and shellfish – as these all contain particularly high amounts of phosphate.

In general, patients only need to worry about the amount of phosphate in their diet if their doctor or dietitian specifically tells them they have a problem.

POTASSIUM

Potassium is another very important mineral in the human body. The kidneys normally regulate potassium levels without any difficulty, but in kidney failure this control is lost. Potassium levels may then be either too high or too low (see *Chapter 11, page 72*).

The main problem with potassium is that if it rises to a very high or a very low level in the blood, then it becomes very dangerous to the heart, which will stop beating.

Potassium is one of the substances that is measured when dialysis patients have blood tests. Any patient who regularly has high blood potassium levels will get to know their dietitian very well. The dietitian will try to find out if the patient is eating anything that might be causing a high level of potassium in the blood.

Many foods contain potassium, but some have more than others. Kidney patients whose blood potassium levels are high or rising will normally be asked to restrict their intake of high-potassium foods. This will involve avoiding some (rather nice) foods, such as chocolate and crisps, and moderating their intake of other potassium-containing foods, such as bananas, oranges and mushrooms.

PD patients rarely need to restrict their potassium intake, and in fact may sometimes need to increase it. This is because PD is a continuous process that generally clears potassium from the blood very effectively. Haemodialysis, on the other hand, is an intermittent process. So, in the intervals between dialysis, the blood potassium may begin to rise. These patients may therefore sometimes need dietary advice on potassium intake.

Unless their doctor or dietitian tells them otherwise, kidney patients can assume that they do not have a problem with their blood potassium.

WHAT ABOUT SALT AND FLUID?

Salt and fluid advice are often given together. A salty diet may make patients thirsty, and make life very uncomfortable if a fluid restriction is necessary.

A salt restriction usually involves:

- using little or no salt in cooking and at the table;
- decreasing the intake of high-salt foods, which are mainly convenience and processed foods.

Haemodialysis patients often have greater restrictions on fluid intake than PD patients, and therefore need to be extra careful about salt.

Fluid advice for individual kidney patients is based on a combination of their urine output (if they still pass urine) and the amount of water removed by dialysis. Generally speaking, the more urine a patient passes, the more fluid they can drink. A common generalisation is that dialysis patients can drink 500–750 mls of fluid every day plus the equivalent of their urine output on the previous day. For many patients, this works out to be about 1 litre for haemodialysis patients and 1.5 litres for PD patients.

VITAMIN SUPPLEMENTS

There are different opinions about the value of vitamin supplements when someone has kidney failure.

Most doctors and dietitians agree that the so-called 'fat-soluble vitamins' (i.e., vitamins A, D, E and K) are rarely a problem and don't need supplementing. Supplements of fat-soluble vitamins may even cause problems, as excessive amounts accumulate in the body. One fat-soluble vitamin – vitamin A (found in large amounts in cod and halibut liver oil capsules) – is known to be toxic and can cause problems if taken to excess.

It is known that the so-called 'water-soluble vitamins' (i.e., vitamins B and C) are lost in both types of dialysis. It is therefore possible that there may be deficiencies if patients reduce their intake of certain foods, either voluntarily or because of potassium restrictions. A case can therefore be made for supplements of these vitamins. But should everyone take supplements, just to make sure (bearing in mind the large numbers of tablets most kidney patients are taking anyway)? Different units adopt different policies.

INDIVIDUAL DIETARY RECOMMENDATIONS

All people with kidney failure are advised, as far as possible, to follow 'Healthy Eating Guidelines' (in brief, to eat a high-fibre, moderate-fat and low-salt diet). In some cases, however, specific individual priorities will over-ride these guidelines.

The most common example of going against the usual guidelines is if someone is losing a lot of weight and needs to boost their intake of calories with fat. In this situation, malnutrition is a more serious and immediate danger than any possible future increased risk of heart disease from a high-fat diet. Hence the reason for the 'unhealthy' compromise on fat intake.

DIET AFTER A TRANSPLANT

A common question after someone has had a kidney transplant is, 'Do I still need to follow a special diet?' The simple answer is, 'No'. If a kidney is functioning well, then there is no need to be on a special diet. If the transplant starts to fail, the situation may be different.

Transplant patients are, however, advised to follow normal 'Healthy Eating Guidelines'. This is particularly important because of two problems associated with a transplant. Both these problems – excessive weight gain (usually a side effect of taking steroid drugs, such as *prednisolone*) and high cholesterol levels – increase the risk of heart disease. Healthy eating habits may help reduce the risk.

KEY FACTS

1. Dietary advice differs according to the stage of kidney failure, and the type of treatment a patient is receiving.
2. 'Healthy Eating Guidelines' – for a high-fibre, moderate fat and low salt diet – are generally recommended whether a patient is pre-dialysis, on dialysis or with a transplant.
3. It is difficult to measure a patient's nutritional state. The blood albumin level is often used, but is not very reliable.
4. Kidney patients should only alter their diet when advised to do so by their doctor or dietitian.
5. Malnutrition is the major problem for many patients on dialysis – both PD and haemodialysis. So, high protein intakes are recommended.
6. Potassium restriction is generally not needed on PD but may be needed on haemodialysis.
7. Excessive salt makes people thirsty. Salt intake may need to be restricted, particularly if fluid is restricted.
8. Most transplant patients will not have any dietary restrictions. They should follow 'Healthy Eating Guidelines'.

13 PSYCHOLOGICAL ASPECTS

This chapter looks at the reasons why people with kidney failure may feel different from healthy people. It also suggests how to identify and cope with the various psychological problems that kidney patients sometimes experience.

INTRODUCTION

Kidney failure has a massive impact on the whole of a person's life – not just on their physical condition. If someone has kidney failure, they have to alter the way they live, to learn new words and skills, and to meet many different people. Kidney failure also affects how people feel about themselves, their sense of purpose, mood, relationships, thoughts and beliefs. The psychological aspects of kidney failure are extremely important.

BODY AND MIND

A kidney patient's psychological and emotional well-being has a major impact on their physical well-being. The way someone feels influences the way they behave. If a person feels low, they may eat or drink to cheer themselves up. If they are anxious, they may row with their partner. If they don't feel able to manage, they may decide their whole treatment is not worth bothering with.

The way a kidney patient behaves has a direct effect on their physical condition. They may become less careful about their diet, or forget to take their tablets, or abandon fluid restrictions – all of which put additional strain on an already poorly body.

PSYCHOLOGICAL NEEDS

Psychology is about behaviour: why people behave the way they do, and how they can change the way they behave. It is about how people feel about themselves, their situation, the people who are part of their lives.

Everybody has psychological needs – not just kidney patients. However old or ill we might be, we all need to be heard, understood and valued. Illness can make this more difficult. When we are unwell, we may find it hard to express our fears and anxieties, and to feel in control of the situation.

STRESSES ON KIDNEY PATIENTS

Kidney failure, being a long-term and life-threatening illness, can be extremely stressful. Any change is stressful, even if it is pleasant, like getting married. But if the changes are 'negative', as when someone has kidney failure, the stresses are greatly increased.

The treatment of kidney failure enforces major changes in life-style. Patients have to adapt their usual routine. They may have to make changes to their eating and drinking habits. They may not have sufficient energy to continue working or to pursue hobbies or interests.

Some of the stresses that commonly affect kidney patients are:

- having to make decisions about things they have never even thought about before;
- taking in strange information, to enable them to understand a complex medical subject;
- learning about themselves and the ways they cope with things;
- needing to ask for support to manage their treatment;
- seeing themselves as a complete person, not just as a disease or condition;
- learning to live differently for the rest of their life;
- worrying about the future.

Changes to the way that life usually progresses may also cause stress. For example, it may be difficult for a young person to leave home, either because they have kidney failure, or because they feel they should look after a parent with kidney failure. Sometimes a kidney patient will have to cope with unpleasant reactions from their employers and work colleagues. Later in life, retirement may come early and be totally unwelcome.

Other members of the family also have to make adjustments. Kidney failure has an impact on their lives too. The normal pattern of family life is disrupted and relationships have to be adjusted.

The diagnosis

For some people, the diagnosis of kidney failure comes completely out of the blue. This can be extremely difficult to cope with. Even when kidney failure was already suspected, confirmation of the diagnosis can cause difficulties. The way that the diagnosis is given, and the quality of support offered immediately afterwards, can make a big difference to a kidney patient's future well-being.

Initial reactions

Following a diagnosis of kidney failure (or any other serious long-term illness), people typically go through the following stages:

1. Shock. At first, patients (and sometimes also family members and friends) go into a state of shock, feeling stunned or bewildered or strangely detached – as though they are observing life rather than being part of it. This shock can last a short while or may continue for weeks.

2. Grief. Then people begin to react to the news, often with feelings of loss, grief, helplessness and despair. They may feel overwhelmed by reality, and find it difficult to think clearly or plan effectively.

3. Denial. One very common reaction to serious illness is to deny the existence of the disease or its implications. But the problem does not go away, the symptoms get worse and there are reminders from other people that the illness exists.

4. Acceptance. Gradually, people come to accept reality a little at a time, and begin to make progress towards adapting successfully to their condition.

Longer-term problems

Patients with kidney failure also often experience longer-term psychological problems. These problems may include:

1. Non-compliance. This is a dreadful doctors' term for 'not doing what you are told'. Common reasons why patients may find it difficult to do as they are told are:
- they believe that the treatment is not effective, and there is no obvious benefit from it;
- they do not know what effect the treatment is supposed to have, or why it is important to continue with it;
- the side effects of the treatment are unpleasant.

Problems with non-compliance can often be solved by better communication between doctors or nurses and their patients.

2. Anxiety. As well as the anxieties felt by most people at some time in their lives, kidney patients also have additional anxieties relating to their condition and its treatment. Some possible problem areas include:
- Relationships:
  'We can't share the same interests any more.'
  'We've both changed so much.'
- Quality of life:
  'I miss walking the dog.'
  'I planned to go abroad.'
- Employment:
  'I've taken too much time off work.'
- Management:
  'How can I do my CAPD exchanges when I feel so ill?'
- Understanding:
  'I can't understand all the medical words.'

3. Body image. Not all kidney patients have problems with their changed body image, but some do. They may see their fistula or PD catheter as a mutilation of their body. They feel horribly scarred and find it really hard to look at themselves.

The perceptions of patients and medical staff can differ widely here. When doctors and nurses talk about a 'really good fistula', they are talking about the ease of access, the rate of blood flow, and the strength of the blood vessels. What the patient experiences is a forearm with a continuous buzzing sensation, and a disfiguring swelling where it used to be smooth and flat. Some patients cannot see their fistula as a 'good' thing at all.

4. Awareness of early death. People with kidney failure know that without treatment they would die. Few people have to live with this sort of knowledge. It puts a totally different perspective on life priorities.

5. Dependency and self-confidence. Kidney patients are very dependent – on hospital doctors and nurses, and on their carers (partners, relatives and friends). People with kidney failure have to deal with the fact that their life depends on a machine, on PD bags, or on someone else's kidney. This necessary dependency can undermine a patient's confidence in coping with both kidney and non-kidney issues:
- 'Am I doing it right?'
- 'I used to take care of her. Now I'm dependent on her.'

If issues relating to dependency and self-confidence are not dealt with, they may cause conflict between kidney patients and hospital staff or carers.

6. Sense of loss. Your kidneys have been a part of you since you were born. For most of your life, like everyone else, you have taken your kidneys for granted, never had to think about them. Now your kidneys have failed, their failure provokes a kind of grieving.

7. Depression. Most people get depressed at some stage in their lives. Periods of depression may be useful, in that they enable people to withdraw from the world for a while, and resolve certain issues. People with kidney failure are no exception. There are times when they feel low, and to do anything at all requires a huge effort; times when they should allow themselves to feel sorry about themselves; and times to cry.

8. Changes to treatment. One of the many difficult things about kidney failure is that the treatment changes over time. For example, patients may change from PD to haemodialysis, or vice versa, or they may receive a transplant, or resume dialysis after a transplant fails.

9. Ageing. It is not only a patient's treatment that changes. Everyone changes to some extent as they get older. Tasks that seem easy when someone is young may become more troublesome as the years go by. Coping with kidney failure may become more difficult.

10. Sexual activity. Sexual problems are very common among people with kidney failure and can put strain on a relationship. Concerns about sexual ability vary from person to person. There may be a loss of sex drive, especially in men. For many young men, the most distressing aspect of kidney failure is their inability to get or maintain a normal erection. For women, there may be worries about getting pregnant, or of having a successful pregnancy. (See *Chapter 14* for more information about sexual problems and their treatment.)

11. Conflicting advice. People with kidney failure receive information from lots of different people. The people who pass on this information have themselves already interpreted it according to their own backgrounds and beliefs. So, what a patient hears may not always be totally true. The advice from one source may conflict directly with advice from another. It is not surprising that kidney patients are sometimes confused by what they are told.

12. Poor concentration. Kidney patients sometimes worry that kidney failure may be affecting their brain. They may find that they sometimes cannot concentrate as well, or think as clearly, as they used to before they developed kidney failure. These problems may last from a few minutes to several days at a time. However, for most people with kidney failure, most of the time, the ability to concentrate and think clearly is as good as it ever was. When there are problems, efficient dialysis will often help a patient to think straight.

FACTORS AFFECTING THE ABILITY TO COPE

Some people cope more easily than others with the psychological and emotional aspects of kidney failure. Research indicates that an individual's ability to cope with illness is influenced by a range of factors.

1. Illness-related factors. The first group of factors relates to the illness itself.

- Some patients are more afraid than others of the possible consequences of kidney failure. Fears of possible disability, disfigurement, pain or early death may need to be addressed. The more a patient feels threatened by their illness, the harder they will find it to cope.
- Kidney failure often occurs together with other conditions, such as diabetes, anaemia (see *Chapter 5*) and renal bone disease (see *Chapter 6*). These conditions cause their own symptoms, giving kidney patients even more things to worry about.
- Some kidney patients have to cope with unpleasant side effects from their medications.
- The treatment of kidney failure involves major time commitments, which can make it difficult for patients to find or hold down a job. Lack of secure employment is an additional strain.
- Kidney failure requires patients and their families to make changes in their life-styles. These changes may put pressure on relationships and increase stress.
- Many people with a chronic illness, such as kidney failure, feel self-conscious about their disease and

want to hide it from others. This can cause stress and make it harder to cope.

2. Age. The age at which a person develops kidney failure is an important influence on how they will cope.

- Children are unlikely to be capable of fully understanding the condition and its long-term implications.
- Adolescents need to be liked and accepted by their peers. Because of this, some of them neglect their medical care to avoid appearing different from their friends.
- In early adulthood, people with kidney failure may resent not having had the chance to develop their lives in the direction they planned – to get married, to have children or to enter a particular career.
- Middle-aged patients may have problems adjusting to the disruption of an established life-style and to being unable to finish tasks they have started, such as building up a business.
- In old age, patients may resent not being able to enjoy their retirement.

3. Personality. Aspects of a patient's personality can affect their ability to cope with kidney failure.

- People who cope well with long-term health problems tend to have hardy or resilient personalities which allow them to see good in difficult situations. They are able to balance hope against despair and to find purpose in life whatever happens. They maintain their self-esteem and resist feeling helpless and hopeless.
- Kidney failure often means that the patient must initially take on a dependent and passive role. Some people find this especially difficult since it is so different from the independent role they have developed over the years.

4. Social and cultural factors. A person's ability to cope with illness is also affected by their background.

- People from different social, cultural and religious backgrounds will have different ways of dealing with things. Problems may arise if doctors and nurses fail to take this into account.
- Peoples' beliefs about health come from a number of sources, including the media, advertising and their friends. These beliefs may be incorrect or only half true. Sometimes, misconceptions can add to the difficulties in adjusting to kidney failure. For instance, people who believe that nothing is seriously wrong unless they are in pain are not likely to seek help for a condition that has no obvious symptoms, such as high blood pressure.

5. Support. The amount and quality of support available to patients are further influences on how well they cope with kidney failure.

- People who live alone, away from their family and with few friends tend to adjust poorly to long-term diseases. Other forms of support are particularly important for these people.
- For many kidney patients, the immediate family is the main source of psychological support. For others, this role is taken by one or more close friends. Such support is usually a big help to the patient. However, it is also true that relatives and friends sometimes undermine effective coping by providing bad examples or poor advice.
- Hospitals do not always provide kidney patients with the support they need. The hospital is often a dull place for patients, thereby further depressing their mood. Unfortunately, at present, very few renal units include a clinical psychologist. However, there is a general recognition of the need to provide patients with psychological support, and some nurses have had special training in counselling.
- For some people, lack of practical support at home

may be a problem. Patients may have difficulty getting round their house or doing every-day tasks, and may lack equipment that could help them become more self-sufficient.

- Many support groups have been set up by and for people with kidney failure. These groups can provide emotional and sometimes financial support, as well as information. (See the *Useful Addresses* section at the back of this book, *page 114*.)

COPING STRATEGIES

People with kidney failure use different strategies to help them cope with this long-term illness. Many kidney patients find the following strategies helpful.

- **Denial.** In the early stages, it can be very useful to deny the situation or not to take it seriously. This helps kidney patients to escape from the feeling of being overwhelmed by the disease. It also allows time to organise other, better ways of dealing with the situation. The belief that a person with kidney failure is still the same as everyone else is a very important element in psychological well-being.

- **Information seeking.** People often find it helpful to seek information about their disease and its treatment. Becoming expert in a subject gives people a sense of control over it.

- **Disease management.** Patients also gain a sense of control over their disease by becoming involved in its management – including being responsible for tablet taking and perhaps doing their own dialysis.

- **Prioritising activities.** For some people with kidney failure, it can be helpful in the long term to reduce the importance of some of their current activities, such as social drinking or playing contact sports.

- **Goal setting.** A very useful coping strategy for many people is to set themselves appropriate goals. These might include, for example, exercising or going out, and trying to maintain regular routines.

KEY FACTS

1. Kidney failure has a major impact on the whole of a patient's life.
2. Psychology is about behaviour and beliefs.
3. People with kidney failure have to cope with extra stresses.
4. Kidney failure and its treatment affects the lives of people who live with the patient.
5. People diagnosed with kidney failure usually go through shock, grief, and denial before acceptance.
6. Longer-term problems may involve non-compliance, anxiety, problems with body image, loss of self-confidence, depression, adapting to changes, and a loss of interest in sex.
7. Kidney failure can sometimes affect a person's ability to concentrate and think clearly. Efficient dialysis helps most people.
8. Many factors affect a person's ability to cope with kidney failure.
9. Various coping strategies can help people deal with the psychological problems that often occur with kidney failure.

14 SEXUAL PROBLEMS

This chapter describes the sexual problems commonly experienced by men and women with kidney failure. It examines the causes of these problems, and suggests what can be done about them.

INTRODUCTION

Most people with kidney failure are troubled by sexual problems. Sometimes these problems start quite early in kidney failure, before dialysis is needed. Some patients may then experience an improvement in their sex lives when they start dialysis, but others notice no difference. Other patients with kidney failure develop sexual problems only after they start dialysis (either peritoneal dialysis or haemodialysis). A kidney transplant often improves a person's sex life, but problems may persist. Some kidney patients never have sexual problems.

INVESTIGATING SEXUAL PROBLEMS

In the past, many health professionals working with kidney patients have tended to avoid getting involved with their patients' sexual problems. Patients, doctors and nurses have often been embarrassed to discuss the subject. Even now, despite the more general interest and openness about sexual matters, kidney patients may still find that they have to raise the subject first.

Another possible reason why some doctors and nurses have avoided the subject of sexual problems has been a mistaken belief that the available treatments were unlikely to work. This view needs to be updated.

As with other aspects of kidney failure, there isn't usually just one straightforward problem that can be easily corrected. Often there are several issues to look at, and patience is required. Nevertheless, treatment is usually successful, provided both partners are keen to have a sex life and are willing to accept help.

IMPOTENCE: THE MALE SEXUAL PROBLEM

Men with kidney failure have a variety of sexual problems. These include having sex less often, loss of interest in sex (sometimes called loss of libido), and being unable to ejaculate ('come'). However, the most common sexual problem – and usually the most worrying for the man – is difficulty in getting or keeping a hard penis (erection problems). This is usually called impotence. Erectile dysfunction (ED) is an alternative name.

What normally happens first in men with kidney failure is that they become less able to keep an erection for as long as usual, although they are still able to ejaculate. Eventually, many kidney patients lose the ability to get a hard penis at all. This can obviously lead to frustration, particularly if the sex drive is unchanged. The situation can be even more upsetting if the man's partner interprets the problem as a loss of interest in them personally.

WHAT CAUSES IMPOTENCE?

Impotence has many possible causes. In most men with kidney failure, sexual problems do not have just one cause, but are usually due to a combination of:

1. Poor blood supply. In order to make the penis hard, extra blood enters the penis and is then prevented from leaving it. Many kidney patients have narrowed blood vessels all over their body, including those vessels that supply the penis. This reduces the blood supply to the penis, and makes it difficult to get an erection. It is not just kidney patients who have this problem. It also occurs as part of the natural ageing process and is commoner in older men, as well as in men with diabetes.

2. Leaky blood vessels. To keep the penis hard, the extra blood that has entered the penis must stay inside it. In men with kidney failure, the extra blood sometimes leaks back out of the penis, and so the erection is lost.

3. Hormonal disturbances. Hormones are chemical messengers that control many body functions. They are carried around the body in the blood. Some hormones are specifically designed to control sexual urges. The levels of these sex hormones can be either higher or lower than normal in people with kidney failure. In particular, the testicles may produce less of the male sex hormone, testosterone.

4. Nerve damage. The nerves that supply the penis are also involved in getting an erection. When someone has kidney failure, nerve damage may prevent the nerves from working properly.

5. Tablets. Most tablets do not cause impotence on their own. However, a few drugs can contribute to sexual problems. The biggest culprits are the blood pressure tablets called beta-blockers, such as *atenolol, propanolol, metoprolol* and *bisoprolol*.

6. Tiredness. Tiredness can affect sexual performance. Tiredness in kidney patient may be caused by anaemia (see *Chapter 5*), by under-dialysis (see *page 113*), or by other medical problems, such as heart problems.

7. Psychological problems. When a kidney patient starts dialysis there are many stresses to deal with (see *Chapter 13*). Not surprisingly, some patients feel quite depressed. If so, they may not feel like having sex.

8. Relationship difficulties. The illness of one partner naturally causes stresses in a relationship. For instance, household jobs, such a decorating or washing-up, which

The normal erection process

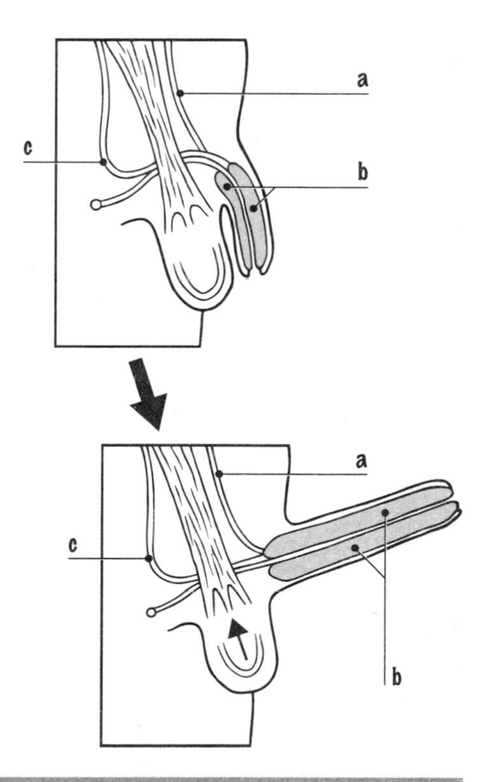

Signals from nerves supplying the genitals cause the main artery of the penis (a) to widen. Extra blood enters the spongy areas of the penis (b) making them swell. The swelling squeezes the veins that carry blood from the penis (c), trapping blood in the penis and making it swell even more

used to be done by the patient may now sometimes have to be done by the partner. This can lead to arguments or resentment on either side of the relationship.

HOW IS IMPOTENCE INVESTIGATED?

The first and most important step is for the subject to be raised. There is often a lot of unnecessary suffering due to either denial of the problem or fear of embarrassment. Some kidney doctors and nurses have no experience of treating sexual problems in people with kidney failure, or are embarrassed themselves. If this is the case, patients should ask to see an expert in sexual problems. Sadly, few kidney units have such an expert at present.

Once the problem of impotence has been recognised, the following should take place:

1. A general health check. This will include an assessment of the distance a person can walk on level ground without having to stop, which is a useful guide to general health.

2. Physical examination. This will include an examination of the genitals. The doctor will also feel for a pulse at various points in the legs. If the pulses are weak, this means that the blood vessels in the legs have narrowed, reducing the blood supply. Then there will usually also be narrowing of the blood vessels supplying the penis, reducing its blood supply.

3. Blood tests. In addition to the usual blood tests, there will be tests to measure the blood levels of various hormones. These include testosterone, and also luteinising hormone (LH), follicle-stimulating hormone (FSH) and prolactin. LH and FSH are hormones that regulate the testicles. Prolactin's usual role is to produce milk in females, but it is often present in larger than normal amounts in male dialysis patients with impotence.

4. Review of medication. The doctor should review the various tablets that the patient is taking. Some types of tablets may contribute to a patient's sexual difficulties. Alternative medication is sometimes available.

5. Investigation of psycho-sexual problems. The patient will be asked to consider whether psychological or relationship difficulties may be contributing to the physical problem of impotence.

HOW IS IMPOTENCE TREATED?

The doctor will begin by looking at any more general problems that may be contributing to a patient's impotence. These may include:

- treating anaemia (see *Chapter 5*);
- increasing the amount of dialysis;
- changing the patient's tablets.

More specific physical treatments for impotence will then be considered. These may include:

- hormone injections;
- use of a vacuum device;
- penile injection therapy;
- penile insertion therapy (transurethral therapy);
- penile implants.

In addition to the various physical treatment options (see *below* for more details), patients may be recommended to seek help for emotional problems relating to impotence (see *below, page 97*).

HORMONE INJECTIONS

Most male dialysis patients with sexual problems have lowish testosterone levels. This deficiency can be treated by an injection of testosterone every three to four weeks. Although testosterone injections replace the hormone that is lacking, they are not always very effective in treating impotence. This is probably because impotence in men with kidney failure is not usually due only to low testosterone levels.

Many other hormones are also often found to be at the wrong level, but correcting them rarely makes much difference to sexual difficulties. If the prolactin level is too high, a tablet called *bromocriptine* (or sometimes one of the newer alternative drugs, such as *cabergoline*) may be given.

VACUUM DEVICES

Many kidney patients with impotence require therapies which act directly on the penis, helping them to get and keep an erection. One of these is called vacuum tumescence therapy, which uses a mechanical device (such as the ErecAid) to produce a hard penis. Nearly three-quarters of the male dialysis patients who use a vacuum device are able to have full penile erections.

To use the vacuum device, the man first inserts his penis into the clear plastic cylinder. He then holds the device against his body so that the chamber is closed with an air-tight seal. Using either a hand- or battery-operated pump, the man then withdraws air from the cylinder to form a vacuum. This causes the penis to enlarge in a way that is similar to a natural erection. However, to maintain the erection, the man must then push a tension ring (resembling an elastic band) from the outside of the cylinder onto the base of the penis. The seal of the vacuum is broken, and the cylinder and pump are removed. With the tension ring in place, the erection can be maintained for up to 30 minutes.

The erections may be longer lasting than natural ones, and do not usually disappear after an orgasm. The most common complaints are mild discomfort and 'timing difficulties' (such as pumping too rapidly with the hand-pump) when the device is first used. Occasionally, harmless, tiny reddish spots (called petechiae) may appear on the penis.

The main advantages of vacuum therapy are that it is safe and non-surgical, can be used as often as desired, and works well for most male dialysis patients. Its suppliers also claim that it may improve blood flow to the penis and result in occasional natural erections.

The disadvantages of vacuum therapy are that it involves a loss of spontaneity in lovemaking, it requires some skill to use, and it can cause mild bruising. It is

An ErecAid

1 The man's penis is inserted into the plastic cylinder of the ErecAid. The ErecAid is then held against the body to form an airtight seal

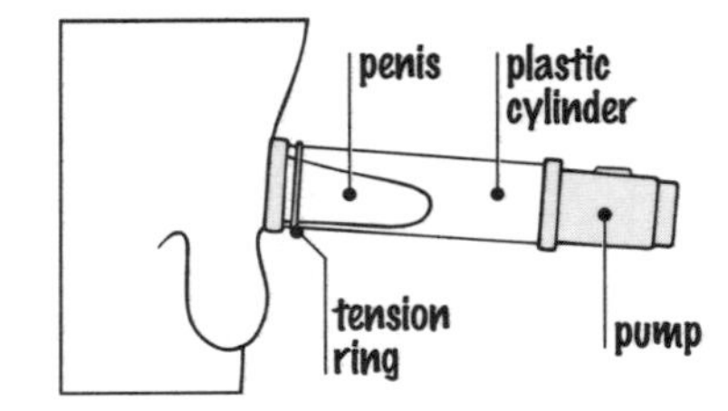

2 The man uses the pump to withdraw air from the cylinder forming a vacuum. The penis enlarges in a similar way to a natural erection

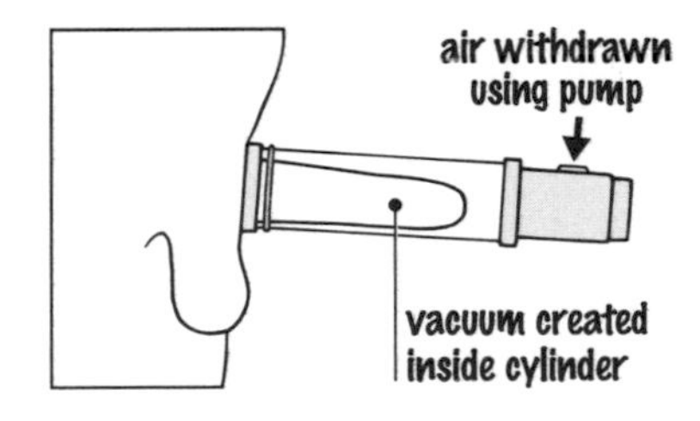

3 The tension ring is slipped off the ErecAid onto the base of the penis to help maintain the erection, and the ErecAid is then removed

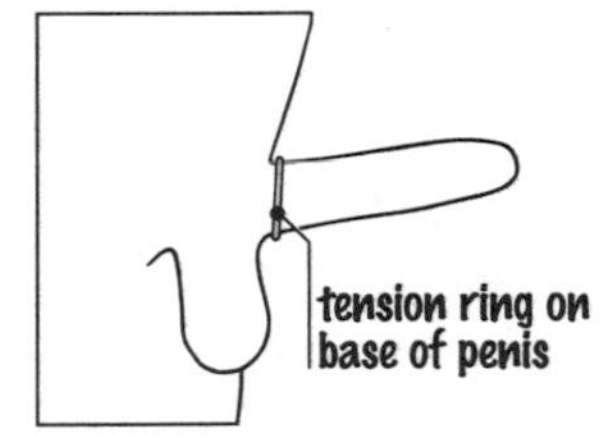

also not available on the NHS. The current cost is about £250, but only the initial outlay is usually required.

PENILE INJECTION THERAPY

Penile injection therapy is another non-surgical technique used to treat impotence. The man injects medication (usually *alprostadil*) into the base of his penis. This causes the penis to become hard almost immediately. The erection then lasts for up to one to two hours.

Use of the injections is limited to not more than once a day and three times a week. Several clinic visits are usually needed to establish the dose of medication required. The treatment is available on the NHS. (The cost is £10 per injection – i.e., typically £500 to £1,000 per year.)

Penile injections have the advantage of not involving surgery. They are also effective in many dialysis patients. It is not known, however, whether the success rate for these injections in kidney patients is as high as the 70% recorded for men who do not have kidney failure.

The main problems with this technique are pain in the penis, and a condition called priapism, which is an unwanted erection that goes on too long. There may also be bleeding, bruising or scarring (fibrosis) at the injection site. Because of the risk of bleeding, patients on haemodialysis are advised not to have the injection on a dialysis day. Another problem is that the penis may become mis-shaped. After a while, some patients get fed up with this treatment, but it is usually possible for them to change to a different therapy option.

PENILE INSERTION (TRANSURETHRAL) THERAPY

This treatment has been available since early 1998 and is proving popular as it is less invasive and intrusive than other physical treatments currently available. As yet, it has been used by only a small number of kidney patients.

For penile insertion therapy, such as MUSE (Medicated Urethral System for Erection), the patient slowly inserts an applicator into the end of his penis. A button on the applicator is then pressed to release a tiny pellet of medication (*alprostadil*). Once the pellet has been released, the applicator is removed and an erection develops over the next 10 to 30 minutes.

Penile insertion therapy has been shown to be successful in just over half the men treated in the general population. The most common side effects are penile discomfort and burning, and light-headedness. Female partners have occasionally reported vaginal burning or itching.

Penile insertion therapy is likely to have a slightly higher failure rate than vacuum devices and penile injections. Nevertheless it is a safe, well-tolerated treatment option. It is available on the NHS, at a cost of about £10 per insertion (the same as penile injection therapy).

PENILE IMPLANTS

The decision to have a penile implant should be made only after very careful consideration. This surgical treatment for impotence is usually effective, but it does have disadvantages (see *below*). Penile implants are available on the NHS, and cost from around £3,000.

The implant is inserted during an operation performed under a general anaesthetic. There are various different types available. Typically, a cylinder implanted in the penis is connected by a tube to a pump in the scrotum. This pump is connected by another tube to a fluid-containing reservoir in the abdomen. Squeezing the pump with the fingers causes fluid to pass from the reservoir into the cylinder, so simulating an erection. The main disadvantage is that the operation to insert the implant alters the penis permanently, ending all hope of natural erections. There is also a risk of infection, and a possibility that the implant will be rejected by the immune system (the body's defence system). Another problem is that an implant can be difficult to conceal.

EMOTIONAL PROBLEMS

Even though the treatments described above usually help to correct erection difficulties, they cannot by themselves restore a sexual relationship.

Sexual problems involve two people, and both partners need to work hard to sort them out. It is very common for people to experience changes in loving relationships after the development of kidney failure. Often, early in kidney disease, one partner becomes the 'carer' and the other adopts the 'sick role'. Later, the improved health of a patient on dialysis, and the desire to restore a sexual relationship, can create new stresses which may take time and patience from both partners to resolve.

Other hidden fears may also be present. For instance, some people may believe that kidney disease could be transferred during sex. This is not true.

Many kidney patients and their partners may want to have counselling, either by a psychologist or sexual counsellor. This can be very effective.

VIAGRA (SILDENAFIL)

Viagra is a tablet treatment for impotence, which has been widely reported in the media since its US launch in April 1998. Viagra acts by enhancing the action of a compound called nitric oxide, which opens wide the blood vessels of the penis, leading to an erection.

Trials of Viagra in diabetic patients with impotence showed that the drug worked in about 50% of these men. The reported side effects were occasional headaches, indigestion, and muscle aches. Patients with angina or other heart problems should not take Viagra.

A recent research study has shown that Viagra works well in up to 75% of PD patients.

SEXUAL PROBLEMS IN FEMALE PATIENTS

Whilst the sexual difficulties of male dialysis patients are often neglected, those of female patients are almost completely ignored. As yet, there has been very little research carried out into the sexual difficulties of female dialysis patients.

The largest study was a survey of 99 Italian female haemodialysis patients. Compared to women who did not have kidney failure, the dialysis patients had sex less often and were less able to have an orgasm. Also, most patients noticed a loss of sex drive.

MENSTRUAL PERIODS AND FERTILITY

It is common for the menstrual periods to become irregular when women develop kidney failure. If a woman with kidney failure does not yet need dialysis, she will probably be less fertile (less likely to become pregnant, even if she is having regular sex) than normal. However, she should use contraception, as pregnancy is still possible.

In dialysis patients, the periods often stop completely. This means that women on dialysis are very unlikely to become pregnant. However, again, women should not rely on this as a form of contraception. It is still possible to get pregnant even if the periods are absent.

Treatment with erythropoietin (EPO) has been shown

to restore menstrual periods in about 50% of women on dialysis. This is thought to be due to two effects of EPO. It improves disturbed hormone levels, and it treats anaemia (see *Chapter 5*). Treatment with EPO increases a woman's chance of becoming pregnant, so contraception should always be used to avoid an unwanted pregnancy.

PREGNANCY AND KIDNEY FAILURE

Becoming pregnant can be hazardous to both mother and baby. The main risk is that the mother will develop very high blood pressure and have a miscarriage.

If a woman with kidney failure wants to try to have a baby, it is better for her to become pregnant before rather than after she starts dialysis. A successful pregnancy is usually possible if the woman's blood creatinine (see *Chapter 2*) is still fairly low (say, less than 200 μmol/l). However, a pregnancy during the early stages of kidney failure may make it necessary to start dialysis sooner than would otherwise have been the case.

There are many problems for women who become pregnant after the start of dialysis. The success rate for pregnancies among women on dialysis is somewhere between 40 and 50 per cent. There is a much better chance of success if a woman is able to wait until after she has had a kidney transplant (particularly if she waits for at least six months after the operation).

KEY FACTS

1. Sexual difficulties affect the majority of male and female dialysis patients.
2. Patients may find that doctors and nurses are reluctant to talk about sexual problems.
3. Impotence (difficulty in getting or keeping a hard penis) is the most common and worrying problem for male patients.
4. Treatment of impotence is usually successful, although patience may be required.
5. Treating anaemia, adjusting the amount of dialysis, and changing tablets can all help.
6. Viagra tablets have been shown to be effective in many dialysis patients.
7. Penile injection therapy may be successful, although there are disadvantages.
8. Penile insertion (transurethral) therapy is a recent advance, but with a slightly lower success rate.
9. Sex counselling can be helpful.
10. Kidney failure affects the periods. Pregnancy is less likely but contraception is still needed.
11. If a woman with kidney failure gets pregnant, there are serious risks to both mother and baby.
12. A successful pregnancy is sometimes possible.
13. If a woman with kidney failure wants to get pregnant, it is best to do so either in the early stages of kidney failure or after a transplant.

15 THE TREATMENT SHORT-FALL

This final chapter compares the rates of kidney failure treatment (dialysis and transplantation) in the UK with similar rates elsewhere in Europe. It also looks at the effect on a patient's life expectancy of kidney failure due to different causes.

INTRODUCTION

The number of patients being treated for kidney failure in the UK has increased in recent years. There is, however, still a serious national shortfall in the provision of both dialysis and transplantation. A comparison with other European countries shows that the UK is well down the international 'kidney treatment league tables'. Far fewer patients in the UK are being treated by dialysis or transplantation than might be expected from the size of the UK population. More money is urgently needed to prolong and improve the lives of many more people with end-stage renal failure (ESRF) in this country. Without dialysis or a transplant, anyone with ESRF will die within a few weeks. With successful treatment, some people with ESRF can expect to live for many years.

EUROPEAN COUNTRIES COMPARED

The kidney treatment league tables included in this chapter are based on statistics obtained from the European Renal Association–European Dialysis and Transplant Association (ERA–EDTA). This organisation, which is based in London, was set up with the following aims:

- to compare the facilities for the treatment of kidney failure in the different European countries;
- to assess and compare aspects of the medical health of patients with kidney failure in the different European countries;
- to find out which patients with kidney failure are more likely to die despite treatment, and when, and why.

Statistics from the ERA–EDTA are the best available indicators of the current provision of kidney failure treatment in different European countries. Although the latest available statistics are for 1995, there is no reason to believe that the overall picture is very different at the time of writing.

Some countries are clearly better than others at reporting their dialysis and transplantation rates to the ERA–EDTA. The UK has a particularly poor record, with only 76% of its specialist renal units sending information to the ERA–EDTA. Better reporting by UK renal units would result in some improvement in the position of the UK in the international kidney treatment league tables, but the UK would still be well down the list. It is impossible to deny the serious under-provision of kidney failure treatment facilities in this country.

In order to make useful comparisons concerning the provision of kidney treatment in different countries it is necessary to take population size into account. This is done by dividing yearly totals from a particular country by the number of millions of people in that country's population. This provides us with tables of comparable figures expressed as numbers per million population (pmp).

The league tables included in this chapter make no allowance for any possible differences in the susceptibility of different national populations to developing kidney failure. For the sake of simplicity, and in the absence of more detailed research, it can be assumed that European national populations are broadly similar with regard to kidney failure. (In fact, countries, such as the UK, that have significant numbers of Black and Asian inhabitants, can generally be expected to have higher numbers of people with kidney failure per million population.)

TAKE-ON RATE FOR DIALYSIS

A useful way of assessing how well (or badly) different countries are meeting their people's need for kidney failure treatment is to use a statistic called the 'take-on rate for dialysis'. This measures the number of new patients per million population who start dialysis in any particular year. A quick glance at the 'European Dialysis League' table (see *right*) reveals that the take-on rate for dialysis in some countries is much higher than in others.

In health care, as in football, some countries are clearly better than others. If all football teams were equally good, all teams would gain the same number of points each year – and all would come 'equal top'. In the UK, Crystal Palace would be as good as Manchester United ... year in, year out. If the health services of all countries

EUROPEAN DIALYSIS LEAGUE

Positions in this league are determined by each country's dialysis take-on rate, i.e., by the number of new patients per million population who started dialysis in 1995.

Position	Country	Take-on rate
1	Germany	163
2	Luxembourg	155
3	Czech Republic	143
4	Italy	131
5	Portugal	126
6	Spain	121
7	Belgium	116
8	Austria	115
9	France	112
10	Sweden	99
11	Denmark	98
12	UK	87
13	Bulgaria	84
14	Netherlands	82
15	Norway	80
16	Hungary	77
17	Greece	75
17	Switzerland	75
19	Ireland	69
20	Finland	68
21	Poland	44
22	Iceland	33
23	Romania	26

were equally good at detecting and treating new patients with kidney failure, the dialysis take-on rate would be the same in all countries, and all their health services would be 'equal top'.

However, not everyone can be top of the league. All European countries do not have the same dialysis take-on rate. One possible explanation for this is that European peoples are not similar – that Romanians, for example, do not often develop kidney failure. This seems unlikely. A much more plausible explanation is that some countries are better than others at identifying and providing treatment for people who develop kidney failure.

There is another reason why some countries – notably Norway, Denmark and Sweden – did not do better in the 1995 'European Dialysis League'. In these countries, it is relatively common for people with ESRF to be given a transplant without ever starting dialysis (see *page 103* for details).

DIALYSIS TAKE-ON IN THE UK

It is very obvious from the 'European Dialysis League' table for 1995 (see *previous page*) that the UK's performance in terms of take-on for dialysis leaves a lot to be desired. The UK came only 12th, with only half the dialysis take-on rate of the top country, Germany. If dialysis were football, the UK would be fighting to stay in the Premier League.

Fortunately for kidney patients in the UK, the national take-on rate for dialysis is improving. In 1995, the UK took on 87 new dialysis patients per million population. This was significantly better than the take-on rate of only 61 in 1993. The provision of dialysis in the UK continues to improve, but the rate of improvement is still far too slow.

The fact that countries such as Germany have much higher dialysis take-on rates than the UK clearly shows that the UK is failing to treat large numbers of people who develop kidney failure. This is all the more worrying when it is remembered that people with ESRF die within a few weeks unless they are treated by dialysis or a transplant.

Not only is the UK's take-on rate for dialysis lower than that in many other European countries, it is well below the level of 150 patients per million population which research suggests is a minimum requirement. The stark reality is that nearly half of the patients who develop ESRF in the UK receive no treatment for it.

PROVISION OF RENAL UNITS

One reason why the provision of dialysis in the UK is so low is the fact that this country has relatively few renal units (and therefore relatively few specialist renal doctors, renal nurses and dialysis machines). A look at the 'European Renal Facilities League' table for 1995 (see *next page*) finds the UK only one place from the bottom of the league, just above Romania.

The actual number of renal units in the UK in 1995 was 83 (compared to 776 in Germany and 654 in Italy). Most UK renal units are based in large cities, which means that many patients have to travel 1-2 hours three times a week for haemodialysis. This means that each of their '4 hour' dialysis sessions actually takes up to 8 hours. In many other countries, even small towns have their own dialysis facilities.

Why does the UK have so few renal units? Not surprisingly, the answer is money. The National Health Service is inadequately funded. The UK needs to put more money into healthcare in general, and into kidney medicine in particular (at present only 1% of the

EUROPEAN RENAL FACILITIES LEAGUE

Positions in this league are determined by the number of renal units per million population in each country in 1995.

Position	Country	Renal units per million
1	Luxembourg	12.5
2	Italy	11.3
3	Germany	9.5
4	Portugal	8.4
5	Greece	8.2
6	Czech Republic	7.7
7	Sweden	7.2
8	Bulgaria	7
9	Switzerland	7
10	Austria	6.8
11	Spain	6.6
12	Belgium	6
13	Hungary	5.5
14	Slovakia	5.2
15	Finland	5.1
16	France	4.7
17	Norway	4.6
18	Poland	3.6
19	Iceland	3.3
20	Netherlands	3.3
21	Denmark	2.9
22	Ireland	1.4
23	UK	1.4
24	Romania	1.1

healthcare budget is spent on treating kidney failure). Then there would be more renal units, more specialist doctors and nurses, more patients dialysed and more transplants performed.

RATE OF TRANSPLANTATION

Another way of assessing how well different countries are meeting the need for treatment for kidney failure is to compare the number of kidney transplants performed per million population in any one year. Like the take-on rate for dialysis (see *page 100*), the rate of kidney transplantation should be the same in all countries. Again, it is easy to see from the 'European Transplant League' table (see *next page*) that this is clearly not the case. Some countries perform many more kidney transplants per million population than others.

The UK has an even worse record in the 'European Transplant League' than in the 'European Dialysis League'. In 1995, the UK came 15th, with 25 transplants per million population. This was lower than in 1994, when the UK was 11th with 30 transplants per million population. The UK clearly has a long way to go before it matches the performance of the two 'European Transplant League' leaders, Norway and Spain.

The 'European Transplant League' table makes no distinction between cadaveric transplants and transplants from living donors. It is worth noting, however, that the countries that do best in this league are those that perform a high percentage of transplants from living donors. In Norway and Sweden, for example, 50% of kidney transplants are from living donors, compared to fewer than 10% in the UK. In 1995, ERA–EDTA data shows that Norway performed 11.9 transplants before dialysis, per million population, followed by Denmark (5.0), Sweden (3.7) and Germany (1.8). The equivalent figure for the UK was only 0.9.

European Transplant League

Position in this league is determined by the number of people per million population who received a kidney transplant in 1995.

Position	Country	Number
1	Norway	56
2	Spain	45
3	Portugal	38
4	Sweden	37
5	Switzerland	36
6	Austria	35
7	Finland	33
7	Luxembourg	33
9	Ireland	32
10	Germany	30
11	Netherlands	29
12	Belgium	28
12	Denmark	28
12	France	28
15	UK	25
16	Italy	24
17	Czech Republic	23
18	Iceland	20
19	Bulgaria	15
20	Greece	14
21	Poland	10
22	Romania	5

Cadaveric transplants in the UK

One reason why the UK does not come higher in the European Transplant League is that this country has a relatively low death rate from road traffic and industrial accidents. This obviously has an effect on the availability of cadaveric kidneys for transplantation. The situation would be improved if more people registered their willingness to donate their organs for transplantation and discussed their wishes with their next of kin.

Even more important is the lack of beds in Intensive Care Units (ICUs) in the UK. If a patient becomes brain dead, and therefore a potential kidney donor, that person needs to be kept on a life-support machine to preserve their organs (including their kidneys) until an operation can be performed to remove them. When ICU beds are in short supply, patients who have a chance of recovery must be given priority over patients who are already brain dead. Inevitably, many potential cadaveric organs are lost in this way. Again, a lack of investment in the National Health Service is an important factor.

Living donor transplants in the UK

It is well worth looking at why the UK carries out so few living related (and unrelated) transplants, especially as this is the best and cheapest treatment for ESRF.

One possible reason why a patient may not be given a living related transplant is that they have no medically suitable donors among their family members. In fact, medical unsuitability among family members is quite uncommon (as proved by the high percentage of living related transplants performed in Norway).

Carrying out a living related or unrelated transplant requires a lot of preparation work by renal doctors, nurses and transplant co-ordinators. Not all renal units in the UK put much time and effort into such work, finding it generally 'easier' (less work) to put patients on the 'normal' (cadaveric) transplant waiting list. Also, by not carrying out transplants from living people, doctors and nurses can avoid having to confront 'difficult' issues with patients and their relatives.

The low rate of transplantation from living donors in the UK is partly the fault of the doctors and nurses who don't always tell patients and their relatives, partners and friends about the full range of possibilities. If potential donors are not told that kidney donation is a possibility, and are not gently encouraged to come forward, they are unlikely to do so. Members of the UK public must also share some of the blame. More relatives, partners and friends need to come forward to donate their kidneys.

SURVIVAL ON DIALYSIS

Age at start of dialysis (in years)	Percentage chance of surviving for 5 years after starting dialysis
Under 15	86%
15-24	86%
25-34	80%
35-44	69%
45-54	57%
55-64	46%
65-74	31%
Over 75	19%

SURVIVAL WITH KIDNEY FAILURE

Before the introduction of dialysis and transplantation, everyone who developed ESRF died within a few weeks. Successful treatment now gives people with ESRF a new lease of life, sometimes for many years.

The 'Survival on Dialysis' table (see *above right*) is based on ERA–EDTA data. It shows the percentage chances of still being alive five years after the start of dialysis. People who start dialysis in younger age groups clearly have a higher percentage chance of surviving for five years than is the case for people who start dialysis later in life. This is not really surprising, given that increased age also reduces the survival chances of people who do not have kidney failure. It remains true, however, that people on dialysis have less chance of surviving for five years than is true for their age group as a whole.

WHY DO PEOPLE WITH KIDNEY FAILURE DIE?

Although people with chronic kidney failure have a lower than average life expectancy, kidney failure is not often fatal. Few people actually die either from kidney failure, from the underlying causes of kidney failure or from treatment for kidney failure (dialysis or a transplant).

People do, however, die from the complications of kidney failure, especially those affecting the heart. It seems that permanent damage to the heart often occurs early in kidney failure, before dialysis or a transplant is needed. This damage is probably due to several factors, including high blood pressure, anaemia and fluid overload. It is also possible that the wastes that build up in the blood in people with kidney failure have a directly toxic effect on the heart. Neither dialysis nor a transplant can do anything to repair an already damaged heart.

DIFFERENT CHANCES OF SURVIVAL

The 'Survival on Dialysis' table (see *above*) provides a useful quick guide to the five-year survival chances of patients starting on dialysis at different ages. However,

Comparative Survival Chances on Dialysis

Percentages of men and women surviving 5 years after the start of dialysis (according to age at the start of dialysis and the cause of end-stage renal failure)

Men

Age (years)	0-14	15-24	25-34	35-44	45-54	55-64	65-74
Cause of ESRF							
Unknown cause	74	85	73	73	63	51	67
Glomerulonephritis	85	84	76	76	68	55	69
Pyelonephritis	84	90	82	73	62	53	69
Polycystic kidneys	84	82	76	63	74	n.a.*	n.a.
Renovascular disease	87	80	72	62	48	62	n.a.
Diabetes	57	55	44	36	28	53	n.a.

Women

Age (years)	0-14	15-24	25-34	35-44	45-54	55-64	65-74
Cause of ESRF							
Unknown cause	74	85	79	76	68	56	39
Glomerulonephritis	84	84	81	77	69	60	43
Pyelonephritis	84	88	84	75	66	57	38
Polycystic kidneys	88	85	78	70	55	n.a.	n.a.
Renovascular disease	75	79	72	64	50	35	n.a.
Diabetes	60	56	46	33	26	23	n.a.

* No data available

age is not the only factor that affects an individual's chances of survival. The table included on this page (again based on ERA–EDTA data) allows some more detailed comparisons.

It can be seen from the table that the sex of patients can sometimes affect their chances of surviving five years after starting dialysis. Under the age of 35 years, there is little difference between the sexes. Over the age of 35, however, women have a slight advantage over men – unless diabetes is the cause of kidney failure, in which case there is no difference between the sexes.

The percentage chance of surviving five years after the start of dialysis is also affected by the cause of kidney failure. Patients with polycystic kidneys have the best chance of survival. They are followed by patients with kidney failure due to glomerulonephritis, pyelonephritis and kidney failure of unknown cause (all of which have similar survival rates). Patients with kidney failure due to diabetes and renovascular disease have the worst survival chances, especially in the older age groups. This is probably because heart attacks and strokes are more common in these patients.

Research has shown that various factors reduce the survival chances of patients on dialysis (or with a transplant). These factors include: a history of a previous heart attack or stroke, peripheral vascular disease (narrowing of the arteries to the legs), serious cancers (including myeloma), diabetes and a rare condition called amyloidosis. If someone with kidney failure has none of these conditions, they have a good chance of long-term survival, either on dialysis or with a transplant.

INDIVIDUALS NOT STATISTICS

Although statistics can give an indication of the average survival chances of different groups of patients treated for kidney failure, they cannot predict what will happen to any one person. People with kidney failure are individuals not statistics. Even if you belong to a group of patients whose overall chance of survival is poor, you as an individual may still survive for many years. Your survival odds are obviously better if you belong to one of the groups with the best chances of survival.

KEY FACTS

1. There is a serious shortfall in the provision of treatment for kidney failure in the UK.
2. Some European countries treat a far higher proportion of their people who develop kidney failure than do others.
3. The UK's yearly 'take-on rate' for dialysis is much lower than it should be. In 1995, the UK was 12th in the 'European Dialysis League'
4. Inadequate funding of the NHS means that the UK has fewer renal units per million population than most other European countries.
5. The UK compares even worse in terms of its yearly transplantation rate. In 1995, the UK was 15th in the 'European Transplant League'.
6. The UK transplants very few patients before dialysis.
7. The UK does comparatively few transplants from relatives, partners and friends.
8. Without dialysis or a transplant, people die within a few weeks of developing ESRF. Successful treatment (by dialysis or a transplant) can prolong life for many years.
9. Average survival chances for people on dialysis (or after a transplant) are affected by age, sex, the underlying cause of kidney failure and various other medical factors.
10. People with kidney failure are individuals not statistics.

GLOSSARY

This glossary provides brief explanations of the various technical words and abbreviations used in this book. Words printed in italic type have their own glossary entry.

Abdomen The lower part of the trunk, below the chest. Commonly called the tummy or belly.
Access A method of gaining entry to the bloodstream to allow *dialysis*. Access methods used for *haemodialysis* include a *catheter, fistula* or *graft*.
Acute A word meaning short-term and of rapid onset, usually requiring a rapid response.
Albumin A type of *protein* that occurs in the blood.
ALG Abbreviation for anti-lymphocyte globulin, a strong treatment against the *rejection* of a *transplant kidney*.
Alkali A substance that is the chemical opposite of an acid.
Alphacalcidol A *vitamin D* supplement.
Amino acids Substances from which *proteins* are built up.
Anaemia A shortage of *red blood cells* in the body, causing tiredness, shortage of breath and pale skin. One of the functions of the *kidneys* is to make *EPO* (erythropoeitin), which stimulates the *bone marrow* to make blood cells. In *kidney failure*, EPO is not made and anaemia results.
Ankle oedema An abnormal build-up of fluid under the skin around the ankles. It is an early sign of *fluid overload*.
Antibiotic drugs A group of drugs used to treat infections caused by *bacteria*.
Antibodies Substances that normally help the body to fight infection. They are made by *white blood cells*. After a *transplant*, antibodies can attack the new kidney and cause *rejection*.
Antigen A type of *protein* that occurs on the outer surface of all the *cells* in a person's body. Antigens act as a 'friendly face' for the cells. The *immune system* normally recognises the friendly face of the body's own cells and does not attack or reject them.
APD Abbreviation for automated peritoneal dialysis. A form of *peritoneal dialysis* that uses a machine to drain the *dialysis fluid* out of the patient and replace it with fresh solution. APD is usually carried out overnight whilst the patient sleeps.
Arteries *Blood vessels* that carry blood from the heart to the rest of the body.
Arteriogram A type of X-ray that uses a special dye to show the blood vessels. The dye is put into the blood vessels via a tube that is inserted into the groin and passed up to the *kidneys*.
Artificial kidney Another name for the *dialyser* or filtering unit of a *dialysis machine*.
ATG Abbreviation for anti-thymocyte globulin, a strong treatment against the *rejection* of a *transplant kidney*.
Atheroma Deposits of *cholesterol* and other fats that cause furring and narrowing of the arteries (also called atherosclerosis).
Azathioprine An *immuno-suppressant drug* used to prevent the *rejection* of a *transplant kidney*.
Bacteria A type of germ. Bacteria are microscopically tiny, single-celled organisms capable of independent life. Most are harmless, but some cause disease.
Beta-blockers Tablets that slow down the heart rate and lower *blood pressure*. Examples are atenolol, metoprolol and propranolol.
Bicarbonate A substance that is normally present in the blood which is measured in the *biochemistry blood test*. A low blood level of bicarbonate shows there is too much acid in the blood.
Biochemistry blood test A test that measures the *blood levels* of various different substances. Substances measured in people with *kidney failure* usually include *sodium, potassium, glucose, urea, creatinine, bicarbonate, calcium, phosphate* and *albumin*.
Biopsy A test involving the removal of a small piece of an *organ* or other body *tissue* and its examination under a microscope.
Bladder The organ in which *urine* is stored before being passed from the body.
Blood cells The microscopically tiny units that form the solid part of the blood. There are three main types: *red blood cells, white blood cells* and *platelets*.
Blood group An inherited characteristic of *red blood cells*. The common classification is based on whether or not a person has certain *antigens* (called A and B) on their *cells*. People belong to one of four blood groups, called A, B, AB and O.
Blood level A measurement of the amount of a particular substance in the blood, sometimes expressed in *mmol/l* (millimoles per litre) or µmol/l (micromoles per litre) of blood.

Blood pressure The pressure that the blood exerts against the walls of the *arteries* as it flows through them. Blood pressure measurements consist of two numbers. The first shows the *systolic blood pressure*, the second, the *diastolic blood pressure*. One of the functions of the *kidneys* is to help control the blood pressure. In *kidney failure*, the blood pressure tends to be high.
Blood vessels The tubes that carry blood around the body. The main blood vessels are the *arteries* and *veins*.
Bone marrow The 'runny' part in the middle of some bones, where *blood cells* are made.
BP Abbreviation for *blood pressure*.
Brain death A term indicating that the entire brain has permanently stopped working, and that further life is possible only on a life-support machine. A person must be diagnosed brain dead before their organs can be removed for a *cadaveric transplant*.
Cadaveric transplant A *transplant kidney* removed from someone who has died.
Calcium A mineral that strengthens the bones. It is contained in some foods, including dairy products. It is stored in the bones and is present in the blood. The *kidneys* normally help to keep calcium in the bones. In *kidney failure*, calcium drains out of the bones, and the level of calcium in the blood also falls.
Candida albicans A fungus that sometimes causes *peritonitis* in patients on *peritoneal dialysis*.
CAPD Abbreviation for continuous ambulatory *peritoneal dialysis*. A continuous form of PD in which patients perform the exchanges of *dialysis fluid* by hand. The fluid is usually exchanged four times during the day, and is left inside the patient overnight.
Catheter A flexible plastic tube used to enter the interior of the body. A catheter is one of the *access* options for patients on *haemodialysis*. For patients on *peritoneal dialysis*, a catheter allows *dialysis fluid* to be put into and removed from the *peritoneal cavity*. A *catheter* may also be used to drain urine from the bladder.
Cells The tiny units from which all living things are built up. Most cells have some common features (including a nucleus that is the cell's control centre and an outer membrane or skin that gives the cell its shape). Cells in different parts of the body look different from each other and perform different functions (for example, skin cells are very different from *blood cells*).
Cholesterol A *lipid* (fat) that is a major contributor to *atheroma*.
Chronic A word meaning long-term and of slow onset, not usually requiring immediate action.
Clearance The removal of the toxic waste products of food from the body. Clearance is one of the two main functions of the *kidneys*. In *kidney failure*, clearance is inadequate and toxins from food build up in the blood.
CMV Abbreviation for *cytomegalovirus*.
Creatinine A waste substance produced by the muscles when they are used. The name creatinine is also given to a blood test that measures the *blood level* of creatinine. The higher the blood creatinine level, the worse the *kidneys* (or *dialysis* or a *kidney transplant*) are working.
Cross-match The final blood test before a *transplant operation* is performed. It checks whether the patient has any *antibodies* to the *donor kidney*. The operation can proceed only if the cross-match is negative (i.e., no antibodies are found).
CT scan Abbreviation for a computerised tomography scan. An investigation that uses a computer to build up a picture from a series of low-intensity X-rays.
Cyclosporin An *immuno-suppressant drug* used to prevent the *rejection* of a *transplant kidney*.
Cytomegalovirus (CMV) A *virus* that normally causes only a mild 'flu-like' illness. In people with a *kidney transplant* (and in other people whose *immune system* is suppressed), CMV can cause a more serious illness, affecting the lungs, liver and blood.
Dehydration A condition in which the body does not contain enough water to function properly. Dehydration often occurs with low *blood pressure*, which causes weakness and dizziness.
Diabetes mellitus A condition (also known as sugar diabetes or simply as diabetes) in which there is too much sugar in the blood. Whether this type of diabetes is controlled by insulin, tablets or diet, it can cause *kidney failure*. This happens most often to people who have had diabetes for longer than ten years.
Dialyser The filtering unit of a *dialysis machine*. It provides the *dialysis membrane* for patients on *haemodialysis*. The dialyser removes body wastes and excess water from the blood in a similar way to a normal *kidney*.
Dialysis An artificial process by which the toxic waste products of food and excess water are removed from the body. Dialysis therefore takes over some of the work normally performed by healthy *kidneys*. The name dialysis comes from a Greek word meaning 'to separate' – i.e., to separate out the 'bad things' in the blood from the 'good things'.
Dialysis fluid The liquid that provides the 'container' into which toxic waste products and excess water pass during *dialysis* for removal from the body.
Dialysis machine The machine used to perform *haemodialysis*.

It includes a *dialyser*, which filters the patient's blood. The machine helps to pump the patient's blood through the dialyser, and monitors the dialysis process as it takes place.
Dialysis membrane A thin layer of tissue or plastic with many tiny holes in it, through which the process of *dialysis* takes place. In *peritoneal dialysis*, the patient's *peritoneum* provides the dialysis membrane. For *haemodialysis*, the dialysis membrane is made of plastic. In each case, the membrane keeps the *dialysis fluid* separate from the blood (essential because dialysis fluid is toxic if it flows directly into the blood). However, the tiny holes in the membrane make it *semi-permeable*, allowing water and various substances to pass through it.
Diastolic blood pressure A *blood pressure* reading taken when the heart is relaxed. It is taken after the *systolic blood pressure* and is the second figure in a blood pressure measurement.
Diffusion A process by which substances pass from a stronger to a weaker solution. Diffusion is one of the key processes in dialysis (the other is *ultrafiltration*). During dialysis, body wastes such as *creatinine* pass from the blood into the *dialysis fluid*. At the same time, useful substances such as *calcium* pass from the dialysis fluid into the blood.
Diuretic drugs The medical name for water tablets. These drugs increase the amount of *urine* that is passed. Two commonly used diuretics are frusemide and bumetanide.
Donor A person who donates (gives) an organ to another person (the *recipient*).
Donor kidney A kidney that has been donated.
Doppler scan A type of *ultrasound scan* (sound-wave picture) that provides information about blood flow through the arteries.
ECG Abbreviation for electrocardiogram. A test that shows the electrical activity within the heart.
ECHO Abbreviation for echocardiogram. A type of *ultrasound scan* (sound-wave picture) that shows how well the heart is working.
End-stage renal failure (ESRF) A term for advanced chronic *kidney failure*. People who develop ESRF will die within a few weeks unless treated by *dialysis* or *transplantation*. These treatments control ESRF but cannot cure it. Once a patient has developed ESRF, they will always have it, even after a transplant.
End-stage renal disease (ESRD) An alternative name for *end-stage renal failure*.
EPO Abbreviation for *erythropoeitin*.
Erythropoeitin A *hormone*, made by the *kidneys*, which stimulates the *bone marrow* to produce *red blood cells*.
ESRF Abbreviation for *end-stage renal failure*.
ESRD Abbreviation for *end-stage renal disease*.
Exit site The point where a *catheter* comes out through the skin. Exit site infections can be a problem for PD patients.
Fistula An enlarged *vein*, usually at the wrist or elbow, that gives *access* to the bloodstream for *haemodialysis*. The fistula is created by a surgeon in a small operation. It is done by joining a vein to an artery. This increases the flow of blood through the vein and causes it to enlarge, making it suitable for haemodialysis needles.
FK506 Another name for *tacrolimus*.
Fluid overload A condition in which the body contains too much water. It is caused by drinking too much fluid, or not losing enough. Fluid overload occurs in *kidney failure* because one of the main functions of the *kidneys* is to remove excess water. Fluid overload often occurs with high *blood pressure*. Excess fluid first gathers around the ankles (*ankle oedema*) and may later settle in the lungs (*pulmonary oedema*).
Glomerulus One of the tiny filtering units inside the *kidney*.
Glomerulonephritis Inflammation of the *glomeruli*, which is one of the causes of *kidney failure*.
Glucose A type of sugar. There is normally a small amount of glucose in the blood. This amount is not usually increased in people with *kidney failure* unless they also have *diabetes mellitus*. Glucose is the main substance in PD fluid, drawing excess water into the *dialysis fluid* from the blood by *osmosis*.
Graft A type of *access* for *haemodialysis*. The graft is a small plastic tube that connects an artery to a vein. It is inserted into the arm or leg by a surgeon. Haemodialysis needles are inserted into the graft, which can be used many hundreds of times.
Haemodialysis A form of *dialysis* in which the blood is cleaned outside the body, in a machine called a *dialysis machine* or kidney machine. The machine contains a filter called the *dialyser* or artificial kidney. Each dialysis session lasts for three to five hours, and sessions are usually needed three times a week.
Haemodialysis catheter A plastic tube used to gain *access* to the bloodstream for *haemodialysis*.
Haemodialysis unit The part of a hospital where patients go for *haemodialysis*.
Haemoglobin (Hb) A substance in *red blood cells* that carries oxygen around the body. *Blood levels* of haemoglobin are measured to look for *anaemia*. A low Hb level indicates anaemia.
Hb Abbreviation for *haemoglobin*.
Heart-beating donor A term used to describe a *donor* whose heart is still beating after *brain death* has occurred. Most, but not all, *cadaveric transplants* come from heart-beating donors.

Hepatitis An infection of the liver, usually caused by a *virus*. Two main types, called hepatitis B and hepatitis C, can be passed on by blood contact. This means that *dialysis* patients, especially those on *haemodialysis*, have an increased risk of getting these infections. Care is taken to reduce this risk, and regular virus checks are made on all kidney patients.
Home haemodialysis Treatment on a *dialysis machine* installed in a patient's own home. For home haemodialysis to be considered, the patient must have a partner or friend who is able to supervise every dialysis session.
Hormones Substances that act as chemical messengers in the body. They are produced in parts of the body called endocrine glands. Hormones travel around the body in the blood and control how other parts of the body work. For example, *parathyroid hormone* from the *parathyroid glands* affects *kidney* function.
Hyperparathyroidism A disorder in which the *parathyroid glands* make too much *parathyroid hormone.*
Intravenous pyelogram (IVP) A special X-ray of the *kidneys*. A dye that shows up on X-rays is used to show the drainage system of the kidneys. The dye is injected into the patient's arm, travels in the blood to the kidneys, and is passed from the body in the *urine.*
Immune system The body's natural defence system. It includes *organs* (such as the spleen and appendix), lymph nodes (including the 'glands' in the neck) and specialist *white blood cells* called *lymphocytes*. The immune system protects the body from infections, foreign bodies and cancer. To prevent *rejection* of a *transplant kidney,* it is necessary for patients to take *immuno-suppressant drugs.*
Immuno-suppressant drugs A group of drugs used to dampen down the *immune system* to prevent *rejection* of a *transplant kidney*. Commonly used examples are *cyclosporin, azathioprine* and *prednisolone*. *Tacrolimus* (FK506) is a newer example.
IVP Abbreviation for *intravenous pyelogram*.
Kidneys The two bean-shaped body *organs* where *urine* is made. They are located at the back of the body, below the ribs. The two main functions of the kidneys are to remove toxic wastes and to remove excess water from the body. The kidneys also help to control *blood pressure*, help to control the manufacture of *red blood cells* and help to keep the bones strong and healthy.
Kidney biopsy Removal of a small piece of *kidney* through a hollow needle for examination under a microscope. It is needed to diagnose some causes of *kidney failure*, including *nephritis*.
Kidney donor A person who gives a *kidney* for *transplantation*.
Kidney failure A condition in which the *kidneys* are less able than normal to perform their functions of removing toxic wastes, removing excess water, helping to control blood pressure, helping to control red blood cell manufacture and helping to keep the bones strong and healthy. Kidney failure can be acute or chronic. Advanced chronic kidney failure is called *end-stage renal failure* (ESRF).
Kidney machine Another name for a *dialysis machine*.
Kidney transplant An alternative name for a *transplant kidney,* or for the *transplant operation* during which a new *kidney* is given to the *recipient*.
LFTs Abbreviation for liver function tests.
Line infection A term for an infection of a *haemodialysis catheter* (or line).
Lipids Another name for fats. People with *kidney failure* tend to have raised lipid levels in the blood.
Liver function tests (LFTs) Blood tests that show how well the liver is working. They often appear at the bottom of the *biochemistry test* results. Some people with *kidney failure* also have liver problems.
Living related transplant (LRT) A *transplant kidney* donated (given) by a living relative of the *recipient*. A well-matched living related transplant is likely to last longer than either a *living unrelated transplant* or a *cadaveric transplant*.
Living unrelated transplant A *kidney transplant* from a living person who is biologically unrelated to the recipient (such as a husband or wife).
LRT Abbreviation for a living related transplant.
Lymphocytes Specialist *white blood cells* that form part of the *immune system*.
Malnutrition Loss of body weight, usually due to not eating enough (especially foods providing protein and energy). Malnutrition is the major nutritional problem of *dialysis* patients.
Marker A substance that is known to occur in the presence of another substance. Both *creatinine* and *urea* are markers for many less easily measurable substances in the blood. The higher the *blood levels* of these marker substances, the higher also are the levels of harmful *toxins* in the blood.
Membrane A thin, skin-like layer, resembling a piece of 'cling film'. The *peritoneum* is a natural membrane used as the *dialysis membrane* in *peritoneal dialysis*. In *haemodialysis,* the dialysis membrane is a plastic membrane inside the *dialyser*.
Methylprednisolone A strong version of *prednisolone,* a drug used to prevent or treat the *rejection* of a *transplant kidney*.
Mmol/l Abbreviation for millimoles per litre. A unit used to measure the *blood levels* of many substances. *Creatinine* is

measured in smaller units called micromoles per litre (μmol/l).
Molecule The smallest unit that a substance can be divided into without causing a change in the chemical nature of the substance.
MRI scan Abbreviation for magnetic resonance imaging scan. A scanning technique that uses magnetism, radiowaves and a computer to produce high-quality pictures of the body's interior.
Nephr- Prefix meaning relating to the *kidneys*.
Nephrectomy An operation to remove a kidney from the body. A bilateral nephrectomy is an operation to remove both kidneys.
Nephritis A general term for inflammation of the *kidneys*. Also used as an abbreviation for *glomerulonephritis* (GN). A *kidney biopsy* is needed to diagnose nephritis.
Nephrology The study of the kidneys.
Oedema An abnormal build-up of fluid, mainly water, in the body. People with *kidney failure* are prone to *fluid overload* leading to oedema. The two most common places for water to collect in the body are around the ankles (*ankle oedema*) and in the lungs (*pulmonary oedema*).
OKT3 Abbreviation for Orthoclone K T-cell receptor 3 antibody, a strong treatment for the *rejection* of a *transplant*.
Organ A part of the body that consists of different types of *tissue* and that performs a particular function. Examples include the *kidneys*, heart and brain.
Osmosis The process by which water moves from a weaker to a stronger solution through tiny holes in a *semi-permeable membrane*. In *peritoneal dialysis*, it is osmosis that causes excess water to pass from the blood into the *dialysis fluid*.
Parathyroidectomy An operation to remove the *parathyroid glands*.
Parathyroid glands Four pea-sized glands near the thyroid gland at the front of the neck. They produce *parathyroid hormone*.
Parathyroid hormone (PTH) A *hormone* produced by the *parathyroid glands*, which helps control *blood levels* of *calcium*. When the level of calcium in the blood is low, PTH boosts it by causing calcium to drain from the bones into the blood. PTH is the best long-term indicator of the severity of *renal bone disease*.
PCKD Abbreviation for *polycystic kidney disease*.
PD Abbreviation for *peritoneal dialysis*.
PD catheter A plastic tube through which *dialysis fluid* for *peritoneal dialysis* is put into, and removed from, the *peritoneal cavity*. The catheter is about 30 cm (12 in) long and as wide as a pencil. A small operation is needed to insert the catheter permanently into the abdomen.
Peritoneal cavity The area between the two layers of the *peritoneum* inside the *abdomen*. The peritoneal cavity contains the abdominal organs, including the stomach, liver and bowels. It normally contains only about 100 ml of liquid, but expands easily to provide a reservoir for the *dialysis fluid* in *peritoneal dialysis*.
Peritoneal dialysis (PD) A form of *dialysis* that takes place inside the patient's *peritoneal cavity*, using the *peritoneum* as the *dialysis membrane*. Bags of *dialysis fluid*, containing glucose (sugar) and various other substances, are drained in and out of the peritoneal cavity via a *PD catheter*.
Peritoneal equilibration test (PET) A measurement of the rate at which *toxins* pass out of the blood into the *dialysis* fluid during *peritoneal dialysis*. Patients are described as 'high transporters' (if the toxins move quickly) and 'low transporters' (if the toxins move more slowly). The test is used to assess a patient's suitability for different types of PD.
Peritoneum A natural *membrane* that lines the inside of the wall of the *abdomen* and that covers all the abdominal organs (the stomach, bowels, liver, etc.). The peritoneum provides the *dialysis membrane* for *peritoneal dialysis*. It has a large surface area, contains many tiny holes and has a good blood supply.
Peritonitis Inflammation of the *peritoneum,* caused by an infection. People on *peritoneal dialysis* risk getting peritonitis if they touch the connection between their *PD catheter* and the bags of *dialysis fluid*. Most attacks are easily treated with *antibiotic drugs*.
PET In this context, an abbreviation for the *peritoneal equilibration test*. (The abbreviation PET in PET scan is short for positron emission tomography.)
Phosphate A mineral that helps *calcium* to strengthen the bones. Phosphate is obtained from foods such as dairy products, nuts and meat. The *kidneys* normally help to keep the right amount of phosphate in the blood. In *kidney failure*, phosphate tends to build up in the blood. High phosphate levels occur with low calcium levels in people with *renal bone disease*.
Phosphate binders Tablets that help prevent a build-up of *phosphate* in the body. Phosphate binders combine with phosphate in food so that it passes it out of the body in the faeces. The most commonly used phosphate binders are calcium carbonate (e.g., Calcichew) and aluminium hydroxide (e.g., Alucaps).
Plasma The liquid part of the blood in which the *blood cells* float.
Platelets A type of *blood cell* that helps the blood to clot.
Polycystic kidney disease (PCKD) An inherited disease (a disease that runs in families) in which both kidneys are full ('poly-'

means 'many') of cysts (abnormal lumps). PCKD is one of the causes of *kidney failure*. It is diagnosed by an *ultrasound scan*.
Potassium A mineral that is normally present in the blood, and which is measured in the *biochemistry blood test*. Either too much or too little potassium can be dangerous, causing the heart to stop. People with *kidney failure* may need to restrict the amount of potassium in their diet.
Prednisolone A drug used to prevent the *rejection* of a *transplant kidney*.
Proteins Chemical components of the body, formed from *amino acids*. The body needs supplies of protein in the diet to build muscles and to repair itself.
PTH Abbreviation for *parathyroid hormone*.
Pulmonary oedema A serious condition in which fluid builds up in the lungs, causing breathlessness. People with *kidney failure* develop pulmonary oedema if *fluid overload* is not treated promptly.
Pyelonephritis Inflammation of the drainage system of the *kidneys,* one of the causes of *kidney failure*. It can be diagnosed by an *ultrasound scan* or by an *intravenous pyelogram* (IVP).
Radio-isotope scan A method of obtaining pictures of the body's interior, also called a radio-nuclide scan. A small amount of a mildly radioactive substance is either swallowed or injected into the bloodstream. The substance gathers in certain parts of the body, which then show up on pictures taken by a special machine.
Radio-nuclide scan Another name for a *radio-isotope scan*.
Recipient In the context of *transplantation*, a person who receives an *organ* from another person (the *donor*).
Red blood cells Cells in the blood which carry oxygen from the lungs around the body.
Reflux The movement of a liquid, such as *urine*, in the opposite direction to normal. The word reflux is sometimes used to mean *reflux nephropathy*.
Reflux nephropathy A condition in which *urine* passes back up from the *bladder*, through the *ureter*, to the *kidney*, where it can cause infections. It occurs because a valve that normally prevents the backflow of urine from the bladder is faulty. Reflux nephropathy is one of the causes of *kidney failure*.
Rejection The process by which a patient's *immune system* recognises a *transplant kidney* (or other transplanted *organ*) as not its 'own' and then tries to destroy it and remove it from the body. Rejection can be *acute* or *chronic*.
Renal Adjective meaning relating to the *kidneys*.
Renal bone disease A complication of *kidney failure*, in which bone health is affected by abnormally low *blood levels* of *calcium* and *vitamin D* and high levels of *phosphate*. Without treatment, renal bone disease can result in bone pain and fractures.
Renal unit A hospital department that treats disorders of the *kidneys*.
Renovascular disease *Atheroma* affecting the *blood vessels* that supply the *kidneys* ('reno-' means relating to the kidney, and '-vascular' means relating to the blood vessels). Renovascular disease is a common cause of *kidney failure* in older patients.
Rigors Cold shivers that sometimes occur with a fever. They can be a symptom of an infected *haemodialysis catheter*.
Satellite haemodialysis unit A place where some patients go for *haemodialysis* away from the main hospital *renal unit*. Satellite units have relatively few nurses and are suitable only for healthy patients, who do some of the haemodialysis preparation themselves. These units tend to be more easily accessible to patients than most main hospital buildings.
Scan One of several techniques for obtaining pictures of the body's interior without using conventional X-rays. Examples include *CT scans, MRI scans, radio-isotope scans* and *ultrasound scans*.
Semi-permeable An adjective, often used to describe a *membrane*, meaning that it will allow some but not all substances to pass through it. Substances with smaller *molecules* will pass through the holes in the membrane, whereas substances with larger molecules will not.
Sodium A mineral that is normally present in the blood, and which is measured in the *biochemistry blood test*. Sodium levels are not usually a problem for people with *kidney failure* and are quite easily controlled by *dialysis*.
Sphygmomanometer The instrument used to measure *blood pressure*.
Staphylococcus One of a group of *bacteria* responsible for various infections (often called 'staph' infections). A common cause of *peritonitis* in patients on *peritoneal dialysis* and of *line infections* in *haemodialysis* patients.
Systolic blood pressure A *blood pressure* reading taken when the heart squeezes as it beats. The systolic blood pressure is measured before the *diastolic blood pressure* and is the first figure in a blood pressure measurement.
Tacrolimus A new *immuno-suppressant drug,* also known as FK506, which may take over from *cyclosporin* as the mainstay of immuno-suppression.
Tissue A collection of similar *cells* that share a similar function, such as skin cells or *kidney* cells.
Tissue type A set of inherited characteristics on the surface of

cells. Each person's tissue type has six components (three from each parent). Although there are only three main sorts of tissue type characteristic (called A, B and DR), each of these comes in 20 or more different versions. Given the large number of possibilities, it is unusual for there to be an exact tissue type match between a *transplant kidney* and its *recipient*. However, the more characteristics that match, the more likely is a transplant to succeed.

Tissue typing A blood test that identifies a person's *tissue type*.

Toxins Poisons. One of the main functions of the *kidneys* is to remove toxins from the blood (a process known as *clearance*).

Transplant A term used to mean either a *transplant kidney* (or other transplant organ) or a *transplant operation*.

Transplantation The replacement of an *organ* in the body by another person's organ. Many different organs can now be successfully transplanted, including the *kidneys*, liver, bowel, heart, lungs, pancreas, skin and bones.

Transplant kidney A *kidney* removed from one person (the *donor*) and given to another person (the *recipient*). Transplant kidneys may be either *cadaveric transplants, living related transplants* or *living unrelated transplants*.

Transplant operation The surgical operation by which a patient is given a donated *organ*. The operation to insert a *transplant kidney* takes about two to three hours. The new *kidney* is placed lower in the *abdomen* than the patient's own kidneys, which are usually left in place. Blood vessels attached to the *transplant kidney* are connected to the patient's blood supply, and the new kidney's *ureter* is connected to the patient's *bladder*.

Transplant waiting list A system that seeks to find the 'right' transplant organ for the 'right' patient. It is coordinated nationally by *UKTSSA*, whose computer compares patients' details (including *blood group* and *tissue type*) with those of cadaveric organs that become available. The average waiting time for a *transplant kidney* is about two years.

Tunnel infection A possible problem for patients on *peritoneal dialysis*. It occurs when an infection spreads from the *exit site* into the 'tunnel' (i.e., the route of the *PD catheter* through the abdominal wall).

UKTSSA Abbreviation for United Kingdom Transplant Support Service Authority, based in Bristol. This is the national coordinator for *cadaveric transplants* in the UK.

ULTRA Abbreviation for Unrelated Live Transplantation Regulatory Authority. This government body must give approval to all *living unrelated transplants*.

Ultrafiltration The removal of excess water from the body. Ultrafiltration is one of the two main functions of the *kidneys*. In *kidney failure*, problems with ultrafiltration result in *fluid overload*. *Dialysis* provides an alternative means of ultrafiltration.

Ultrasound scan A method of obtaining pictures of internal *organs,* such as the *kidneys*, or of an unborn baby, using sound waves. A device that sends out sound waves is held against the body. The sound waves produce echoes, which the scanner detects and builds up into pictures.

Under-dialysis Not having enough *dialysis*. If a dialysis patient doesn't achieve target *blood levels* for *creatinine,* the symptoms of *kidney failure* are likely to return. The amount of dialysis will then have to be increased.

Urea A substance made by the liver. It is one of the waste products from food that builds up in the blood when someone has *kidney failure*. Like *creatinine*, urea is a *marker* for other more harmful substances. The higher the urea level, the worse is the kidney failure.

Ureters The tubes that take *urine* from the *kidneys* to the *bladder*.

Urethra The body's tube that takes *urine* from the *bladder* to the outside of the body.

Urinary catheter A plastic tube inserted into the *bladder* for the removal of *urine*.

Urine The liquid produced by the *kidneys,* consisting of the toxic waste products of food and the excess water from the blood.

Vancomycin An *antibiotic drug*, commonly used to treat *peritonitis* and *line infections*.

Vasodilator drugs Tablets that lower the *blood pressure* by making the blood vessels wider, so that the blood can flow through them more easily.

Veins Blood vessels which carry blood from the body back to the heart.

Virus A type of germ responsible for a range of mild and serious illnesses. Viruses are much smaller than *bacteria* and usually reproduce inside the *cells* of other living organisms.

Vitamin D A chemical that helps the body to absorb *calcium* from the diet. Blood levels of vitamin D are usually low in people with kidney failure.

Water tablets The common name for *diuretic drugs*.

White blood cells Cells in the blood that normally help to fight infection. They are part of the *immune system*. After a *kidney transplant*, they can be a 'bad thing', as they may attack (reject) the new kidney.

Xenotransplantation The transplanting of *tissues* or *organs* from one type of animal into a human or other type of animal.

USEFUL ADDRESSES

The following organisations offer support, information and, in some cases, financial assistance.

Access to Communication & Technology
Oak Tree Lane Centre
Oak Tree Lane
Selly Oak
Birmingham B29 6JA

Tel: 0121 627 8235
Fax: 0121 627 8210

Age Concern England
Astral House
1268 London Road
London SW16 4ER

Tel: 020 8679 8000
Fax: 020 8679 6069
Web: ace.org.uk

Association of Disabled Professionals
170 Benton Hill
Wakefield Road
Horbury
W. Yorkshire WF4 5HW

Tel/Fax: 01924 283 253
email: AssDisProf@aol.com

British Diabetic Association
10 Queen Anne Street
London W1M 0BD

Careline: 020 7636 6112
Tel: 020 7323 1531
Fax: 020 7637 3644
email: bda@diabetes.org.uk
Web: www.diabetes.org.uk

British Kidney Patient Association
Bordon
Hampshire GU35 9JZ

Tel: 01420 472 021
Fax: 01420 475 831

Cancerlink
11-21 Northdown Street
London N1 9BN

Helpline: 0800 132 905
Asian Language Helpline: 0800 590 415
email: cancerlink@canlink.demon.co.uk

Carers National Association
20-25 Glasshouse Yard
London EC1A 4JT

Tel: 020 7490 8818
Fax: 020 7490 8824
email: internet@ukcarers.org
Web: www.carers.demon.co.uk

Department of Health
Richmond House
79 Whitehall
London SW1A 2NS

Tel: 020 7210 4850
Web: www.open.gov.uk/doh/dhhome.htm

Department of Social Security
Disability Benefit Centre
Olympic House
Olympic Way
Wembley
Mddx HA9 0DL

Tel: 020 8795 8820
Fax: 020 8795 8798

Disability Information Trust
Mary Marlborough Centre
Nuffield Orthopaedic Centre
Headington
Oxford OX3 7LD

Tel: 01865 227 592
Fax: 01865 227 596
email: disinfo@sable.ox.ac.uk

Disability Scotland
Princes House
5 Shandwick Place
Edinburgh EH2 4RG

Tel: 0131 229 8632
Fax: 0131 229 5168
email: disability.scotland@virgin.net
Web: dis–scot.gcal.ac.uk

Disability Wales/Anabledd Cymru
Llys Ilfor
Crescent Road
Caerphilly
Mid Glamorgan CF83 1XL

Tel: 029 2088 7325
Fax: 029 2088 8702
email: info@dwac.demon.co.uk

Employment Opportunities for People with Disabilities
123 Minories
London EC3N 1NT

Tel: 020 7481 2727
Fax: 020 7481 9797
Web: www.opportunities.org.uk

Family Fund
PO Box 50
York YO1 2XZ

Tel: 01904 621 115
Fax: 01904 652 625

Family Holiday Association
2nd Floor Rear
16 Mortimer Street
London W1M 7RD

Tel: 020 7436 3304
Fax: 020 7436 3302
Web: www.fhaonline.org.uk

Holiday Care Service
Imperial Buildings
2nd Floor
Victoria Road
Horley
Surrey RH6 7PZ

Tel: 01293 774 535
Fax: 01293 784 647

Lifeline
113 Winston Road
London N16 9LN

Tel/Fax: 020 7254 5245
email: val.said@virgin.net

Medic-alert Foundation
1 Bridge Wharf
156 Caledonian Road
London N1 9UU

Tel: 020 7833 3034
Fax: 020 7713 5653
email: info@medicalert.co.uk

National Kidney Federation
6 Stanley Street
Worksop
Notts S81 7HX

Tel: 01909 487 795
Fax: 01909 481 723
email: nkf@kidney.org.uk
Helpline: 0845 601 0209
Web: www.kidney.org.uk

The National Kidney Research Fund
King's Chambers
Priestgate
Peterborough PE1 1FG

Tel: 01733 704 650
Fax: 01733 704 692
email: enquiries@nkrf.org.uk
Web: www.nkrf.org.uk

Shaw Trust
Shaw House
Epsom Square
White Horse Business Park
Trowbridge
Wiltshire BA14 CXJ

Tel: 01225 716 300
Fax: 01225 716 333

Skill (National Bureau for Students with Disabilities)
Chapter House
18–20 Crucifix Lane
London SE1 3JW

Tel: 020 7450 0620
Fax: 020 7450 0650
email: SkillNatBurDis@compuserv.com
Web: www.skill.org.uk
Freephone: 0800 328 5050
Text: 0800 068 2422

SPOD (Association to Aid the Sexual and Personal Relationships of Disabled People)
286 Camden Road
London N7 0BJ

Tel: 020 7607 8851
Fax: 020 7700 0236

INDEX

In the index, page numbers in bold plain type refer to the glossary, numbers in bold italic type indicate a diagram.

J

K

L

M

N

ORDER FORM

Photocopy this form and send it (post free in the UK) to:

Class Publishing Customer Service
FREEPOST (no stamp needed)
LONDON W6 7BR

Tel: 01752 202301
Fax: 01752 202333

Please send me urgently (tick boxes below)	**Post included price per copy (UK only)**
☐ **Kidney failure explained** (ISBN: 1 872362 90 7)	£17.99
☐ **Food for life** (ISBN: 0 9528823 1 0)	£11.50
☐ **Alzheimer's at your fingertips** (ISBN: 1 872362 71 0)	£17.99
☐ **High blood pressure at your fingertips** (ISBN: 1 872362 81 8)	£17.99
☐ **Diabetes at your fingertips** (ISBN: 1 872362 79 6)	£17.99
☐ **Parkinson's at your fingertips** (ISBN: 1 872362 96 6)	£17.99
☐ **Cancer information at your fingertips** (ISBN: 1 872362 56 7)	£17.99
☐ **Heart health at your fingertips** (ISBN: 1 872362 77 X)	£17.99
☐ **Stroke at your fingertips** (ISBN: 1 872362 98 2)	£17.99
☐ **Stop that heart attack!** (ISBN: 1 872362 85 0)	£17.99
☐ **Asthma at your fingertips** (ISBN: 1 85959 006 3)	£17.99
☐ **Allergies at your fingertips** (ISBN: 1 872362 52 4)	£17.99
TOTAL	

Easy ways to pay

Cheque: I enclose a cheque payable to Class Publishing for £ __________

Credit card: please debit my ☐ Access ☐ Visa ☐ Amex ☐ Switch

Number ______________________ Expiry date ______________________

My address for delivery is ______________________

Name ______________________

Address ______________________

____

Town ______________ County ______________ Postcode ______________

Telephone number (in case of query) ______________________

Class Publishing's guarantee: remember that if, for any reason, you are not satisfied with these books, we will refund all your money, without any questions asked. Prices and VAT rates may be altered for reasons beyond our control.